From Revolution to Rights in South Africa

Dedicated to my late father
Herbert Leopold Robinsky

From Revolution to Rights in South Africa

Social Movements, NGOs
& Popular Politics after Apartheid

STEVEN L. ROBINS
Professor of Social Anthropology
in the University of Stellenbosch

JAMES CURREY

UNIVERSITY OF KWAZULU-NATAL PRESS

James Currey
www.jamescurrey.com
is an imprint of Boydell & Brewer Ltd
PO Box 9, Woodbridge, Suffolk IP12 3DF, UK
and of Boydell & Brewer Inc.
668 Mt Hope Avenue, Rochester, NY 14620, USA
www.boydellandbrewer.com

University of KwaZulu-Natal Press
Private Bag X01
Pietermaritzburg
Scottsville 3209
South Africa
www.ukznpress.co.za

British Library Cataloguing in Publication Data
Robins, Steven L.
From revolution to rights in South Africa: social movements,
NGOs & popular politics after apartheid 1. Social movements
– South Africa 2. Group identity – South Africa 3. Civil
society – South Africa 4. AIDS (Disease) – Political asects
– South Africa 5. Community organization – South Africa
6. South Africa – Politics and government – 1994- 7. South
Africa – Social conditions – 1994-
I. Title
303.4'84'0968

ISBN 978-1-84701-202-9 (James Currey cloth)
ISBN 978-1-84701-201-2 (James Currey paper)
ISBN 978-1-86914-164-6 (University of KwaZulu-Natal Press paper)

Typeset in 10.5/12.5pt Monotype Bodoni by forzalibro designs, Cape Town

Contents

1

Introduction   1
From Revolution to Rights

2

Activist Mediations of 'Rights' & Indigenous Identity   29
Land Struggles, NGOs & Indigenous Rights
in Namaqualand

3

Citizens & 'Bushmen'   51
The ≠khomani San, NGOs,
& the Making of a New Social Movement

4

'Civil Society' & Popular Politics in the Postcolony   77
'Deep Democracy' & Deep Authoritarianism
at the Tip of Africa?

5

AIDS, Science & the Making of a Social Movement   100
AIDS Activism & Biomedical Citizenship
in South Africa

Foreword & Acknowledgements

During the years from 1990 to 1992 I lived in Sengezane village in Gwaranyemba Communal Area in Zimbabwe's Gwanda District in Matabeleland. At the time I was busy doing my doctoral fieldwork on village-level politics of land resettlement and rural development. Quite early on during my fieldwork I visited Zimbabwe's capital city Harare with the intention of conveying to Dr Joseph Made, then a senior manager in the Agricultural Rural Development Authority (ARDA), some of the seething problems I had encountered at ARDA's 'Model D' resettlement scheme in Sengezane village. In good faith, and in retrospect rather naively, I thought that I could convince the ARDA manager to change the top-down, technicist implementation of extremely disruptive land-use planning interventions in Sengezane village. I had seen first hand how these land-use plans had caused havoc with villagers' daily lives and livelihood practices. I had hardly begun to outline the kinds of village-level complications and hardships these plans had unleashed, when Dr Made launched into a tirade against foreign researchers who criticised his government without providing solutions.[1] By the time I left this volatile meeting I had reconciled myself to the reality that my research findings would have no impact, and that Robert Mugabe's ZANU-PF government was not interested in criticism. I was relieved to know that, once I finished my fieldwork, I could return to South Africa to make a contribution to my country's new democracy.

The release of Nelson Mandela in February 1990, and the unbanning of the anti-apartheid liberation movements shortly thereafter, ushered in expectations of democratisation and transformation that had once seemed unimaginable. It was this optimism that I witnessed following the 1994 election of Mandela as the first President of the new South Africa. These heady times were also reflected in the extraordinary vibrancy of civic organisations, NGOs, and new social movements that emerged in a post-apartheid political landscape framed by one of the most progressive constitutions in the world. The proliferation of new political move-

---

[1] As it turned out, Joseph Made was later to become the Minister of Lands, and he was responsible for leading the charge of Robert Mugabe's 'fast track' resettlement programme that began in 2000.

ments included those concerned with the environment, indigenous rights, land, biotechnologies, low-income housing, gay and lesbian issues, housing and HIV/ AIDS. It was within this dynamic political moment that the seeds for this book found fertile ground.

During the early 1990s, I became increasingly interested in the role of popular land struggles in catalysing new forms of identity politics amongst people in the Northern Cape Province who were previously classified as 'Coloured' but were increasingly identifying themselves as San, Grique and Nama (Chapters 2 and 3). This period also witnessed the emergence of new forms of transnational activism initiated by community-based organisations such as the South African Homeless Peoples' Federation (SAHPF) (see Chapter 4). Following President Thabo Mbeki's controversial embrace of AIDS dissident views in 1999, my research began to focus on the ways in which AIDS activism was producing new political subjectivities, identities and practices (see Chapters 5 and 6). AIDS activism quickly became much more than a scholarly interest. Like the Treatment Action Campaign (TAC) activists, I too was outraged that President Mbeki embraced AIDS dissident theories and seemed to be in a state of AIDS denial at a time when five to six million South Africans were living with HIV. I soon found myself confronted with new ethical and intellectual dilemmas and challenges as a South African political anthropologist doing research in the midst of a devastating pandemic.

This interest in political anthropology, and my particular focus on social movements and activism, was not accidental; it reflected my growing political awareness as a white South African of the historical burdens of the twin legacies of colonialism and apartheid. These concerns had emerged in the course of my studies at the University of Cape Town (UCT) in the early 1980s. Although I had developed a gut sense of the systemic injustices of apartheid growing up as the son of a German Jewish refugee in the conservative, middle-class white suburbs of Port Elizabeth, it was my voracious reading of the works of South African sociologists, anthropologists and historians such as Martin Legassick, Harold Wolpe, Jean and John Comaroff, and Shula Marks that provided me with a historically and culturally informed understanding of the emergence of what Marxist theorists referred to as South Africa's particular version of 'racial capitalism' and 'colonialism of a special type'.

My training in political anthropology, and my political education more broadly, had begun in earnest in 1979 in the Department of Social Anthropology at the University of Cape Town (UCT). In the late 1980s, social anthropologists at UCT – Emile Boonzaier, Mamphela Ramphele, Peter Skalnik, John Sharp, Andrew Spiegel, Robert Thornton and Martin West – published a pathbreaking critique of apartheid state discourse in an edited volume called *South African Keywords* (1988). This text provided students like myself with the intellectual tools to unpack and deconstruct the apartheid state's discourses on race, ethnicity, tribe and so on. My understanding of the political situation in South Africa was further deepened by my 1982 Honours research on forced removals in Qwaqwa, an impoverished and overcrowded rural homeland of the South Sotho. It was here that I witnessed first hand the devastating consequences of apartheid social engineering, whereby hundreds of thousands of black South Africans were forcibly removed from 'white South Africa' and dumped in underdeveloped labour reserves. This was my real political and intellectual awakening. After completing my Honours degree, I was fortunate to study at Columbia University (1986–1994) in New York with two pre-eminent political anthropologists, George Bond and Joan Vincent. This training exposed me to broader theoretical questions raised by political anthropology in Africa.

This book is a culmination of ethnographic investigations done over the period of more than a decade. The essays were written during a period of dramatic political transformations in terms of which nothing seemed stable and certain. In recent years this political landscape has become even more uncertain. In December 2007, South Africans, including political pundits, journalists and commentators, were taken by surprise by the dramatic electoral victory of former Deputy President Jacob Zuma's 'camp' at the ANC's Conference at Polokwane in Limpopo Province. Although the polls had indicated that Zuma had considerable support at the ANC branch level, not many pollsters predicted that his 'faction' would take a clean sweep of the top six positions of the ANC party leadership. This constituted a 'palace coup' and a dramatic routing of President Mbeki and his support base. Zuma became President of the ANC, thereby thwarting President Mbeki's attempt to win a third term as president of the ruling party.

The book does not, however, deal with ANC party politics and struggles for political power of the sort that surfaced during the build-up to the December 2007 ANC Conference. Neither does it focus on the role of the trade unions and the SACP in national political life. Instead, it focuses on NGO and social movement activism and popular politics during the post-apartheid period. The case studies on land, housing and AIDS activism and mobilisation were researched and written during a period characterised by the global emergence of new social movements and new forms of identity politics. Although class-based mobilisation in the trade union movement has persisted, the book does not delve into the rich and well-researched field of labour movements. The book has also deliberately avoided analysing the twists and turns of political parties, ballots and procedural democracy, an area of study that has tended to be the domain of political science. Hopefully by focusing quite narrowly on NGOs and social movements, it will contribute towards expanding our understandings of new political discourses, organisations, citizenships and identities.

There are numerous individuals I wish to acknowledge. These include my teachers at University of Cape Town, especially Emile Boonzaier, John Sharp, Andrew Spiegel, Robert Thornton, and Martin West, as well as my Columbia University Professors, George Bond, Joan Vincent and Marcia Wright. The list of colleagues and friends who contributed in a variety of ways to the making of this book is long and includes the following researchers, academics and activists: Ted Bauman, Manmeet Bindra, Joel Bolnick, Sarah Bologne, Chris Colvin, Jean Comaroff, John Comaroff, Roger Chennels, David Chidester, Nigel Crawhall, Ben Cousins, Bill Derman, Brahm Fleisch, Kathy Glover, Thomas Koelble, Thami Maqulana, Shula Marks, Donald Moore, Leo Podlashuc, James Suzman, Kees van der Waal, and

Vivienne Ward. Others who were involved in the publication process include Chris Colvin, Lynn Taylor, and Douglas Johnson. I would also like to thank Jonathan Shapiro for allowing me to use his cartoons. Special thanks are also due to Chris Colvin and Brahm Fleisch for their ongoing intellectual engagement, support and collegiality. Other colleagues I would like to acknowledge at Stellenbosch University, University of Cape Town, and the University of the Western Cape include Brenda Cooper, Bernard Dubbeld, Harry Garuba, Hennie Kotze, Nick Shepherd, Chris Tapscott, Lisa Thompson, John Williams and Cherryl Walker.

The three chapters on AIDS activism and health citizenship benefited from the support and inspiration of a number of people including Zackie Achmat, Andrew Boulle, Ruth Cornick, Andrea Cornwall, Nathan Geffen, Eric Goemarre, Tobias Hecht, Melissa Leach, Lyla Metha, Vinh Kim Nguyen, Akhona Ntsaluba, Phumzile Nywagi and Khululeka, Helmuth Reuter, Herman Reuter, Ian Scoones, Raymond Suttner, Leslie Swartz, Bettina von Lieres, and countless TAC and MSF activists who have been the inspiration for this research. I would also like to thank John Gaventa and numerous other participants in the joint School of Government, University of the Western Cape and Institute for Development Studies, Sussex University project on Citizenship, Participation and Accountability. Finally, I would like to thank Lauren Muller for her consistent support, insights and critical engagement with ideas and debates.

The book is a result of a decade of research and writing, and earlier versions of the chapters were published in the following journals and books:

2008 'Sexual Politics and the Jacob Zuma Rape Trial', *Journal for Southern African Studies* (in press).

2006 From Rights to "Ritual": AIDS activism and treatment testimonies in South Africa', *American Anthropologist*, Volume 108, No. 2 (June): 312–23.

2005 'Housing Activist Networks from Cape Town to Calcutta: A case study of the politics of trust and distrust', in Steinar Askvik and Nelleke Bak (eds), *Trust in Public Institutions in South Africa*. Burlington, VT: Ashgate, pp. 121–36.

2004 '"Long live Zackie, Long live": AIDS activism, science and citizenship after apartheid', *Journal of Southern African Studies*, Volume 30, No. 3, (September): 651–72.

2001 'NGOs, "Bushmen" and Double Vision: The ≠khomani San land claim and the cultural politics of "community" and "development" in the Kalahari', *Journal of Southern African Studies*, Volume 27, No. 4, (December): 833–53.

1997 'Transgressing the Borderlands of Tradition and Modernity: "Coloured" identity, cultural hybridity and land struggles in Namaqualand (1980–94)', *Journal for Contemporary African Studies*, 15 (1): 23–44.

Abbreviations

ALP	AIDS Law Project
APF	Anti-Privatisation Forum
ART	anti-retroviral therapy
ARV	anti-retroviral
AZAPO	Azanian People's Organisation
BEE	Black Economic Empowerment
Contralesa	Congress of Traditional Leaders of South Africa
DOT	Direct Observation Therapy
FJZ	Friends of Jacob Zuma
KGNP	Kalahari Gemsbok National Park
Khululeka	Khululeka Men's Support Group, Gugulethu
KZN	KwaZulu-Natal
MDM	Mass Democratic Movement
MSF	Médecins Sans Frontières
NSMs	New Social Movements
NUM	National Union of Mineworkers
PAC	Pan-Africanist Congress
PD	People's Dialogue
PLWAs	People Living with AIDS
PMA	Pharmaceutical Manufacturers' Association
PMTCT	prevention of mother-to-child transmission
POWA	People Opposing Women Abuse
SABC	South African Broadcasting Corporation
SACP	South African Communist Party
SADC	Southern African Development Community
SADF	South African Defence Force
SAHPF	South African Homeless People's Federation
SANAC	South African National AIDS Commission
SASI	South African San Institute
SDI	Slum Dwellers International
SECC	Soweto Electricity Crisis Committee
STS	Science and Technology Studies

TAC	Treatment Action Campaign
TAN	transnational advocacy network
THO	Traditional Healers Organisation
TRC	Truth and Reconciliation Commission
UCKG	(Brazilian) Universal Church of the Kingdom of God
UDF	United Democratic Front
UNWGIP	United Nations Working Group for Indigenous Peoples
VMx	Victoria Mxenge Housing Scheme
WIMSA	Working Group of Indigenous Minorities in Southern Africa

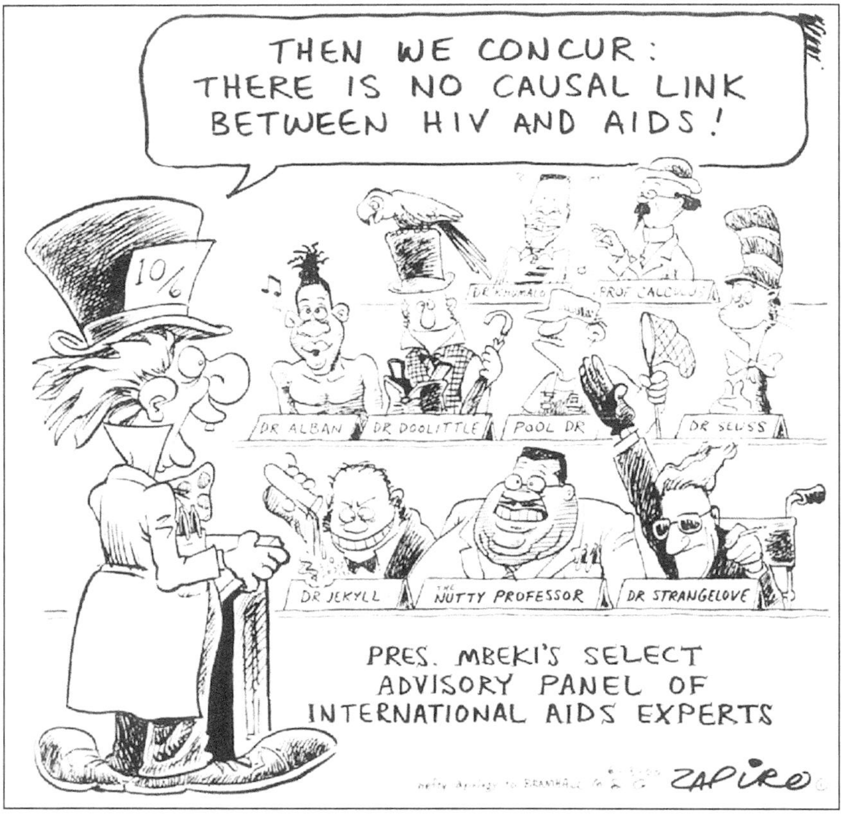

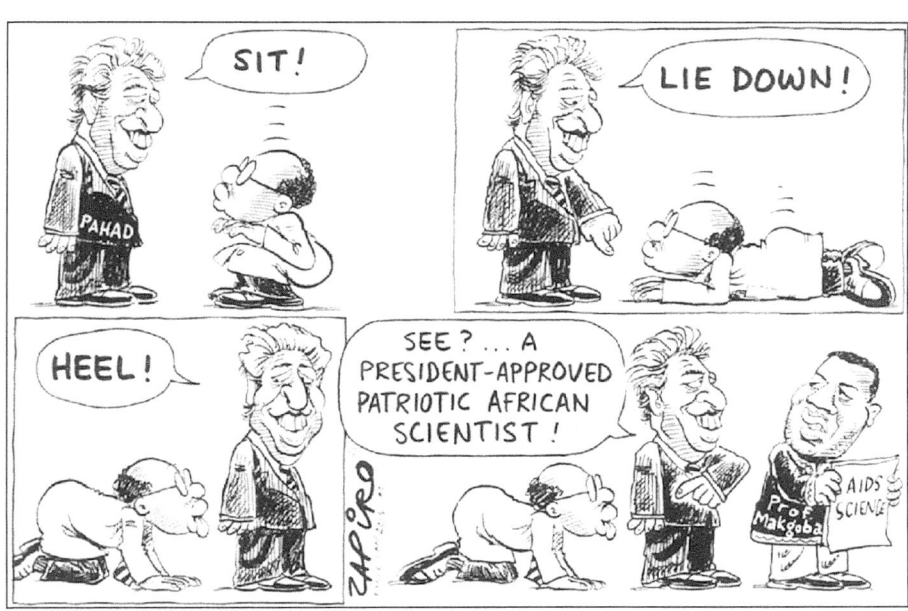

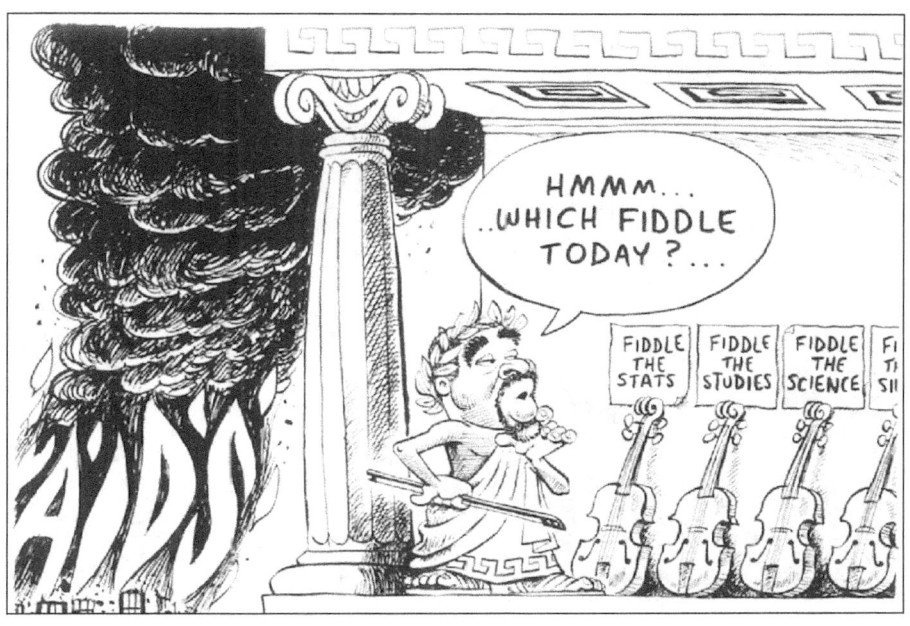

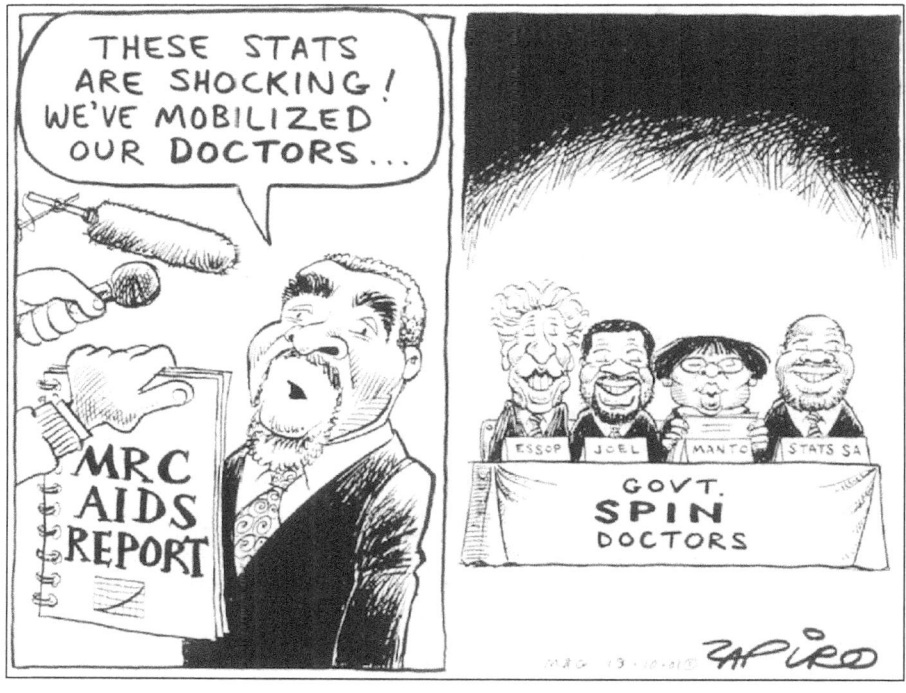

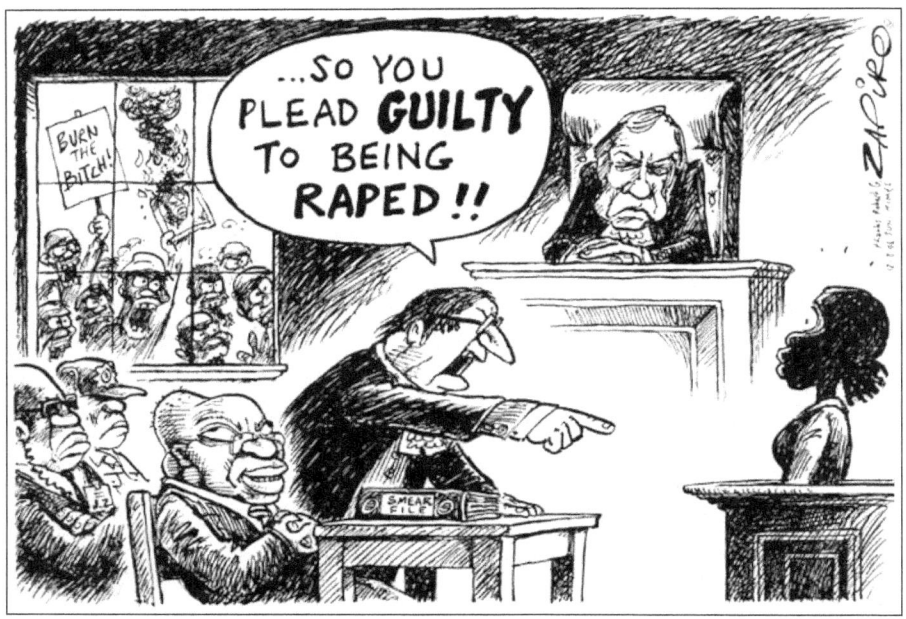

1

Introduction
From Revolution to Rights

We did not say our struggle against apartheid was a civil rights struggle. We said it was a liberation struggle. There is actually a difference ... A liberation struggle includes socio-economic issues, it includes power relations. It includes structures of society, etc. Whereas civil rights is a legalistic notion. For instance, you would agree, surely, if we change the law on the rights of women with respect to property that would not actually emancipate women ... So, when people were talking today, in the [G8 Parliamentary Conference] meeting about women's rights, it was quite a limited, legalistic formulation. (Professor Ben Turok, an African National Congress Member of Parliament, *New Agenda*, Issue 19, 2005:14–15).

Discourses of rights and responsibilities conveniently cast the powers of economy and state as relatively benign at a historical moment when both seem nearly unassailable anyway. (Brown 1995: xiii)

Introduction[1]

During South Africa's first decade of democracy, cultural rights claims took varied and fascinating forms. For example, shortly after the arrival of democracy in 1994, delegations of middle-class white Afrikaners converged on UN-sponsored indigenous rights meetings in Geneva and elsewhere claiming to be indigenous peoples just like the Inuit, the San, Aborigines, Maoris, and so on. At roughly the same time, similarly minded Afrikaners established the all-white *Volkstaat* (Homeland) of Oranje in an attempt to live out their ideals of ethnic self-determination in a post-apartheid constitutional democracy that protected language and cultural rights.

On the other side of the racial divide, in January 2007, animal rights activists from the SPCA contested the right of senior Africa National Congress (ANC) politician Tony Yengeni to spear a bull at a family ritual. Vigorous public debates ensued in the media about Yengeni's 'cruel spearing' of the bull before it was

[1] Acknowledgements – Brahm Fleisch, Chris Colvin, Jean Comaroff, Lauren Muller, Thomas Koelble, Kees van der Waal, Vivienne Ward, Harry Garuba and colleagues at the Centre for African Studies, University of Cape Town.

1

slaughtered at a cleansing ceremony for the four months that he spent in prison for defrauding parliament.[2] In response, Mongezi Guma, the chairman of the Cultural, Religion and Linguistic Rights Commission, claimed that criticism of this age-old Xhosa ritual violated the constitution. As Guma told the press, 'It is ethnocentric and undermining to hide behind animal rights and deny human beings their rights to uphold and practice their cultures and religions. Even more serious is the temptation to violate the constitution, which protects the cultural and religious rights of all who live in South Africa'.[3] Another commissioner, Nokozula Mndende, explained that Yengeni had not speared the bull but merely 'prodded' it with a spear to make the bull 'burp,' or make any other sound, to indicate that the ancestors had accepted the ritual slaughter.[4] Meanwhile, the Ministry of Arts and Culture spokesperson, Sandile Mamela, reiterated the constitution's protection of the right of all indigenous people to perform rituals that connected them with their ancestors.[5] The Minister of Labour, Membathisi Mdladlana, responded by extending an invitation to the Society for the Prevention of Cruelty to Animals (SPCA) 'to join us as we will be slaughtering a bull without [anaesthetizing] it ... We want the bull to bellow – and then we'll sing the praises of our ancestors'.[6] Following initial criticism of these ritually prescribed slaughter methods, the SPCA's executive director, Marcelle Meredith, decided to accept the invitation to attend Mdladlana's ceremony, stating that 'we are assured there is no suffering, if the slaughter is carried out in the traditional manner by a skilled person, taking into account the transport, handling and restraining of the animal'.[7] Clearly, cultural rights, animal rights, and 'rights talk' more generally, have become an integral part of public discourse in the new South Africa. 'Rights' talk has also proven to be sufficiently flexible to be mobilised by widely divergent ends of the political spectrum.

South Africa's relatively peaceful transition to a rights-based constitutional democracy has been praised internationally as a 'miracle'. The larger-than-life figures of former President Mandela and Archbishop Tutu came to embody the possibility of peaceful democratic transitions in even the most violent and conflict ridden societies. South Africa's Truth and Reconciliation Commission (TRC) became a number one export to countries struggling to overcome legacies of violence, brutality, and authoritarianism. Similarly, South Africa's 'state-of-the-art' constitution, with its emphasis on socio-economic, linguistic and cultural rights, as well as and sexual and gender equality, has been touted as one of the most progressive on the planet. However, a decade after democracy the gap has widened between this bright vision of a 'rights paradise' and the grim everyday social, economic and political realities experienced by the majority of South Africa's citizens. This book tracks the twists and turns of 'rights talk' and South Africa's liberal democratic revolution.

2   Vusumuzi Ka Nzapheza, 'Circumstances, not practice of slaughter probed, says SPCA.' *Cape Times*, 24 January 2007, p. 4.
3   '"Yengeni only prodded bull": Cultural panel seeks talks with SPCA on all groups' rites.' *Cape Times*, 26 January 2007, p. 5.
4   Ibid.
5   Ibid.
6   'Mdladlana invites SPCA to witness slaughtering of bull.' *Cape Times*, 29 January 2007, p. 1.
7   'SPCA to see ritual slaughter at Mdladlana's rural home after all.' *Cape Times*, 31 January 2007, p. 3.

Rights, revolution and the limits of liberation

During the course of the ANC's dramatic transformation from liberation movement to ruling party there was a seismic shift in its political lexicon. Radical keywords and concepts such as socialism, national liberation, class struggle, peoples' revolution, resistance to racial capitalism and colonialism-of-a-special type, were replaced with tamer words such as rights, citizenship, liberal democracy, nation-building, transformation, black economic empowerment (BEE) and so on. This dominant language of liberal 'rights' and citizenship is still regularly challenged by the revolutionary rhetoric of the popular Left in the trade union movement and the South African Communist Party (SACP).

Whereas the militant language of national liberation envisioned the revolutionary seizure of state power, the ANC government was soon rudely reminded of the limits of political power in a country characterised by centuries of social and economic inequality and racial domination (Terreblanche 2002). During the anti-apartheid struggle, scholars on the left had described apartheid as a system of racial capitalism whose overthrow would require more than simply taking racially-based legislation off the statute books. Addressing the raw facts of deeply entrenched race and class inequality, it was argued, would require nothing less than a socialist revolution. However, with the collapse of the Berlin Wall and the break-up of the former Soviet Union, socialism was no longer on the cards for a liberated South Africa. These constraints became increasingly visible as the ANC took over the mantle of political power.

This sobering recognition of the limits to liberation after apartheid (Robins 2005) was accompanied by a noticeable shift in the ANC's political ideology and economic programmes. It also involved significant shifts in political language, including the introduction of a new set of liberal democratic keywords. Furthermore, post-apartheid NGOs and social movement activists have increasingly recognised the emancipatory potential of rights-based approaches.

In 2005, a decade after the first democratic elections, Zackie Achmat from South Africa's Treatment Action Campaign (TAC) was nominated for a Nobel Peace Prize. Although the prize was ultimately not awarded to Achmat, his international visibility as the moral voice on HIV/AIDS in the Third World was undisputed. TAC had, since its establishment in 1998, become recognised internationally as one of the most effective AIDS social movements. This was largely due to its dramatic legal victory over the global pharmaceutical industry, which was trying to prevent developing countries from importing and manufacturing antiretroviral generic drugs. Meanwhile, in South Africa, TAC had acquired an equally impressive reputation for its successful court victories and modes of popular mobilisation that eventually compelled a recalcitrant state to provide antiretroviral therapy (ART) to South African citizens living with AIDS (see Chapter 5).

Although post-apartheid South Africa witnessed the emergence of a proliferation of NGOs and social movements in the land, housing, labour and health sectors, amongst others, TAC's innovative forms of rights-based activism captured the imagination of South Africans and international health and development agencies, governments, and civil society organisations.

These new forms of political activism, however, were paralleled by new, sometimes uncomfortable, forms of economic reorganisation. In the same year as Achmat's Nobel nomination, the South African Broadcasting Corporation (SABC) aired the South African version of Donald Trump's franchised reality television show *The Apprentice*. South Africa's home-grown Trump is the revolutionary-turned-billionaire, Tokyo Sexwale. Sexwale, an ex-African National Congress freedom fighter, became one of the country's most wealthy men in the space of a few years following the transition to democracy in the early 1990s. The meteoric rise of former-revolutionaries-turned-corporate elites such as Sexwale and the former trade unionist, Cyril Ramaphosa, reinforced a 'home-grown' ideology of meritocracy that implied that anyone could become filthy rich if they were sufficiently single-minded, talented and determined. In 2007 reports had circulated in the media that Sexwale and Ramaphosa were leading contenders to succeed President Mbeki when he steps down in 2009.

Whereas the liberation struggle mobilised the working class and the 'masses', in the post-apartheid period it appeared that the culture of corporate capitalism rewarded individuals with drive and ability.[8] Black economic empowerment (BEE) initiatives by the new government created opportunities for the extraordinarily rapid accumulation of wealth by a small group of black capitalists. At the same time, however, in a number of speeches in 2006 and 2007, President Thabo Mbeki lashed out against the greed and self-aggrandisement of those who used access to political office and political connections to accumulate personal wealth. In fact, many of the post-apartheid black corporate elites, together with their partners in the state, also preached and promoted the communitarian virtues of the African Renaissance, community development, and *ubuntu*.[9]

This combination of highly individualistic and competitive ideologies of economic liberalism, together with communitarian notions of 'African renewal', resonated in interesting ways with new forms of 'Asian liberalism' which, according to Aihwa Ong (1999: 48), promote both ruthlessly competitive capitalism and developmental programmes initiated by 'caring' and paternalistic Asian states.[10] In other words, rather than seeing the post-apartheid transition as simply a shift to a neo-liberal package of hyper-individualism, 'rights talk' and 'free market' capitalism, it would seem that the political and economic realities reveal a hybrid cocktail comprising both neo-liberal

---

[8] For the South African Left, however, the unimaginable wealth accumulated by this small circle of former anti-apartheid activists is evidence that only a few black South Africans stand to benefit from the transition to liberal democracy (see Bond 2000; Marais 1998). From this perspective, South Africa's particular brand of neoliberal capitalism is characterised by enclaves of extraordinary wealth in a vast sea of racialised poverty and hyper-marginalisation.

[9] *Ubuntu* has come to be understood as an indigenous African philosophy and popular orientation in terms of which people acquire their humanity in relation to others, unlike 'western' forms of liberal individualism and self-interest. It is associated with Nguni-speaking groups and has also been appropriated by consultants who work for business corporations seeking to instil unwavering company loyalty and solidarity that transcends racial and class divides in the workplace. Drucilla Cornell, the philosopher and jurist, is currently involved in an interdisciplinary exploration of *ubuntu*'s ethical, aesthetic and juridical potential in a global context.

[10] Ong, A. 1999. 'Clash of Civilizations or Asian Liberalism? An Anthropology of the State and Citizenship', in Henrietta Moore (ed.), *Anthropological Theory Today*.

features – for instance, privatisation and economic liberalisation policies – as well as discourses of *ubuntu* communitarianism and welfare, housing, land and health programmes typically associated with the African development state.[11]

The corporate capitalist ideology of neo-liberalism and meritocracy did not go down well with all political groupings within the ANC. A decade after democracy, the tensions between President Mbeki's embrace of liberal capitalism – Mbeki Inc. – and the Left's vision of socialist transformation culminated in bruising political battles between supporters of the President and those who lined up behind former Deputy President Zuma. Zuma, who in December 2007 replaced President Mbeki as president of the ANC, was touted as a 'man of the Left' by his supporters within the Congress of South African Trade Unions (COSATU), the South African Communist (SACP) and the ANC Youth League. He was also able to present himself as an African populist and Zulu traditionalist, in stark contrast to the corporate image of President Mbeki as a liberal modernist reformer who promoted sexual and gender equality through gender equity quotas and same-sex marriage laws (see Chapter 7). These leadership conflicts culminated in Zuma's supporters demanding that he should become the next President, notwithstanding President Mbeki's dismissal of Zuma in 2005 from his position as Deputy President following allegations of corruption. This succession crisis split the ANC into pro-Mbeki and pro-Zuma factions, a division that reflected deep ideological rifts within the ANC and its alliance partners, the SACP and COSATU. The succession conflict also revealed some of the deep fissures and contradictions embedded within South Africa's extraordinary transition from apartheid authoritarianism to liberal democracy.

This book is not about these national political developments and conflicts over ANC political ideology, policy and succession. Instead, it focuses more narrowly on how social movements and NGOs have mobilised locally in order to leverage access to state resources such as land, housing and health care. In the process these organisations have strategically engaged with the ANC government, the new rights-based constitutional democracy and global civil society. The case studies are specifically concerned with the dynamics of NGO and social movement partnerships, including how they secure access to state resources by deploying both local rights-based strategies and globally connected modes of collective mobilisation in marginalised communities. These modes of activism, this book argues, reflect a growing trend amongst social movements towards forms of political mobilisation that have been referred to as 'grassroots globalisation' or 'globalisation from below' (Appadurai 2002a, b; Falk 1993). The case studies focus on these twin processes of globalisation and localisation, and investigate how NGO and social movement-mediated forms of popular politics are emerging in these interstitial spaces.

It is an understatement to note that life and politics at the social margins in Africa is a highly uncertain, provisional, and precarious state of affairs. Susan Reynolds Whyte (2002), in a study of AIDS in Uganda, identifies an 'African

---

[11] The Minister of Finance, Trevor Manuel, seemed to make a similar point when he suggested that, contrary to the claims of Left critics, the Growth, Employment and Redistribution (GEAR) macro-economic policy of the ANC government was not part of a fiscally conservative neo-liberal project but was instead the vehicle for realizing the developmental goals of the ANC's Reconstruction and Development Programme (RDP). Trevor Manuel, 'A delicate balancing act'. *Sunday Times*, 13 August 2006, p. 21.

pragmatics' and practical knowledge of everyday life that requires 'trying out alternatives' and opting for provisional solutions (cf. Werbner, 2002: 15). This clearly has implications for the political identities and subjectivities of the poor, as well as for the NGOs and social movements that seek to mobilise them. While rights may be significant and efficacious in settings where there is a relatively well resourced and responsive state, it may make more sense to invest in social networks, clientalistic relations and communal forms of belonging in places where the state is extremely thin on the ground.

In post-colonial contexts like South Africa it makes eminent sense for social actors to speak both the languages of rights and culture. Even traditional leaders resort to 'rights' and litigation to buttress their claims to chiefly rule, property and authority.[12] Warlords and shacklords living in South Africa's shantytowns also draw on rights, as do the crime syndicate kingpins and street gangsters who run Cape Town's multi-billion drug trafficking industry. Rights is increasingly the accepted language of political claims in the new South Africa.

For ordinary citizens, these rights-based approaches are mobilised, often with the help of social movement and NGO activists, to make claims on the state for housing, land, health care and other resources. In other words, rights discourses have been assimilated into popular political culture in post-apartheid South Africa. Yet, although the state is central to the lives of millions of South African citizens, it is not the only game in town. Traditional leaders, clan membership, patron–client relations, religious affiliation and so on, are also extremely important for those living at the margins of the state.

The book focuses on NGO and social movement-driven struggles for marginalised citizens to access land, housing and health care. The case studies show how, in neo-liberal, post-colonial contexts, the poor and marginalised must respond to uncertainty and radical contingencies on a daily basis. This requires multiple strategies – often deployed opportunistically. This suggests an engaged, situated citizenship, one that is linked to daily struggles for survival as well as organised collective mobilisation around rights claimed both at the individual and group level. So how does this 'popular politics' relate to processes of democratisation in post-apartheid South Africa?

In a great deal of the political and academic commentary on the contemporary world order, this kind of complexity and situational strategising is flattened and occluded in favour of a number of simplistic, overarching theoretical propositions. These propositions claim to explain the new historical moment postcolonial citizens in places like South Africa occupy, but the case studies in this book call these propositions into serious question.

Proposition 1 is that we are living in a Post-Cold War, neo-liberal order that spells not only the 'end of history' (Fukuyama 1992), but also an epoch characterised by

---

[12] Former Bantustan traditional leaders of the apartheid era have, for example, become ANC members of Parliament. These former Bantustan traditionalists have also succeeded in pressuring and lobbying the ANC for increased political and land allocation rights, which they claim were guaranteed in terms of the liberal democratic Constitution of post-apartheid South Africa. In South Africa, as elsewhere in the world, traditionalism can be extremely (post)modernist, contingent and strategic. Similarly, political subjectivities are not written in stone but are instead exceptionally plastic and pliable.

'the end of politics', a condition largely associated with neo-liberalism and conditions of hyper-individualisation, voter cynicism, and generalised political apathy in the advanced capitalist countries of the 'overdeveloped' North. *Proposition 2* follows the binary logic of Samuel Huntington's sweeping claims about a Post-Cold War 'clash of civilisations' between the 'Western liberal democracies' and 'Eastern Islamic theocracies'. This clash of civilisations thesis implies a series of binaries that continue to haunt Western popular and scholarly discourses: liberal versus authoritarian; rights versus culture; modern versus traditional; secular versus religious, and so on. *Proposition 3* consists of a widely held view, promoted by political scientists, policy academics, donors and NGOs, that 'civil society' is a space of popular, participatory democracy and horizontal relations of trust and 'positive' social capital. Partha Chatterjee (2004) challenges this uncritical and romantic vision of 'civil society' by arguing that civil society in India, and elsewhere in the Global South, is essentially an enclave of the educated elite that is sequestered from the popular classes, or what he calls 'political society'. While subscribing to some aspects of Chatterjee's critique of conventional ideas about civil society, the book argues that Chatterjee is too sweeping in his characterisation of civil society as an elite enclave. The case studies in this book question the neat analytic separations between the state, civil society and the popular classes that Chatterjee's model implies.

By focusing on new NGO and social movement partnerships that have emerged in South Africa since apartheid, this book interrogates the underlying assumptions of these three propositions. Before surveying the key elements of the argument presented in this book, I will provide a brief overview of the three propositions mentioned above.

Proposition 1: 'The end of politics' (for whom?)

The cover of Zymunt Bauman's (1999) *In Search of Politics* has a photograph of an elderly man sitting alone in a park surrounded by empty benches. This image captures Bauman's bleak assessment of the possibility of re-building public space and collective politics in Europe in a late modern age of rampant privatisation of everyday life. Bauman argues that individual liberty can only be a product of collective work; yet contemporary life in the West is characterised by a movement towards a privatisation of the means to secure individual liberty. Bauman (2001) takes up similar themes in *Community: Seeking safety in an insecure world.* Here the cover consists of a photograph of seven free-falling parachutists holding hands as they plummet towards earth with the last traces of a blood-red sun setting on the horizon. For Bauman, the parachutists represent the hyper-transience of the experimental communities of late modernity – communities built on the freedom to choose to belong and the freedom to terminate membership on short notice. This freedom to 'bail out' at will represents community without long-term commitments. This image is, for Bauman, an illustration of the 'end of (collective) politics' in the advanced capitalist countries of the North.

A number of contemporary political theorists argue that liberal rationalities of government in Europe and North America are contributing towards hyper-individualisation and the depoliticisation of citizens. These processes are seen to be reinforced by new neoliberal forms of governmentality and 'government-at-a-distance' (Barry, Osborne and Rose 1996; Rose 2007; Rose and Novas 2005; Scott 1999). Writing primarily about the UK, Nikolas Rose (1996) argues that in contrast to analyses that stress the reduced role of government within free market economies, neoliberalism governs-at-a-distance by allowing new social actors to become 'subjects of responsibility, autonomy and choice', or what Barry *et al. (*1996) refer to as 'responsibilised citizens'. These new forms of governmentality and biopower are produced through public health discourses, including those promoted by international health agencies, NGOs, social movements and community organisations (Nguyen 2005). They have become particularly powerful sites for the promotion of new forms of self-management and 'therapeutic citizenship' (Nguyen 2005), for example by encouraging citizens to take individual responsibility for preventative health and hygienic measures such as washing one's hands, eating healthily, exercising, practising safe sex and so on (Paley 2002: 483; see Chapters 5 and 6 in this volume). For some critics, these forms of 'governance-at-a-distance' conform to the logic of Tony Blair's 'Third Way' managerialism, and undermine the possibility of radical collective mobilisation.

For some critics of the global hegemony of neoliberal capitalism, liberal democracy and the ubiquitous model of the self-interested and autonomous rights-bearing citizen signal the death knell for collectivist politics. As John Comaroff has remarked, in the contemporary era, class action seems to have replaced class struggle (see also Brown 1995). Similarly, critics argue that liberalism's celebration of the 'freedom to choose' all too seamlessly slides into the 'postmodern' spectre of the depoliticised consumer citizen whose search for meaning and identity is reduced to ceaseless shopping. Marxist intellectuals once understood bourgeois democracy, with its emphasis on individual rights, as an obstacle to true class-consciousness and a socialist utopia that depended on the interventions of vanguard Communist parties and centralised states. With ideas such as class, socialism and revolution virtually absent – or having 'disappeared' – from Post-Cold War academic and popular discourses, 'rights,' 'civil society' and 'citizenship' have become the keywords in both political studies and the donor-driven democracy industry. Yet, as the recent history of trade unionism and the rise of a popular Left in South Africa, Brazil and Latin America shows, revolutionary ideas and grand narratives of socialist transformation continue to animate politics in many parts of the world.

Liberalism's critics also argue that procedural democracy, with its fetishisation of the ballot, 'the law' and multi-party politics, threatens to erase earlier concerns with mass mobilisation, especially those associated with the revolutionary politics of socialist and labour movements. In its place, the 'postmodern turn' has created the conditions for the dizzying proliferation of new identity-based and single-issue social movements that address diverse issues, usually through recourse to the legal system. Wendy Brown (1995) argues that this turn to legal institutions to adjudicate or redress practices of discrimination and social injury threatens to undermine the emancipatory projects of new social movements. What is happening, Brown argues, is the confinement of politics to 'repressive, regulatory and depoliticising [state] institutions that themselves carry elements of the [repressive] regime whose subversion is being sought' (ibid: ix–x).

For critics such as Brown, what appears under the guise of 'progressive politics' is often an embrace of 'litigiousness as a way of political life' (1995: ix). She argues that engaging with 'the law' and liberal discourses of individual rights and responsibilities unwittingly 'increases the power of the state and its various regulatory discourses at the expense of political freedom' (ibid: 28). This turn to the law to regulate and redress social injury, obscures the ways in which domination is reproduced through the double hegemony of capitalism and the state. Brown concludes that disciplinary power is 'extraordinarily effective in "colonising" allegedly free subjects, for example, those highly individuated, self-interested subjects produced by liberal culture and capitalist economics'. It is precisely the belief in their individuation and false autonomy, Brown argues, that renders them so susceptible to disciplinary power (ibid: 19).

Critics of liberalism find that the fragmentation, individualisation and depoliticisation resulting from 'rights talk' and identity politics, together with widespread citizen apathy, have transformed liberal citizenship into the meaningless ritualised act of voting every few years. Yet, even these rituals of liberal democracy are plagued by low voter turnout. Within this 'post-political' and post-socialist world, liberal individualist conceptions of rights might indeed seem to undermine collective forms of emancipatory politics.

This critique of the current moment can also be found in the post-modern turn in social movement theory, much of which argues that new social movements have moved towards increasingly depoliticised and individualist forms of identity politics, thereby fragmenting any possibility of substantive political challenges to structural inequalities, especially those between the North and the South (Edelman 2001).

In recent decades there has been a proliferation of studies celebrating the spectacular growth of globally connected social movements from Seattle to Johannesburg (see Cohen and Rai, 2000). Marc Edelman (2001:285) in an extensive review of the social movements literature, notes that theories of collective action have undergone a number of paradigm shifts from 'mass behaviour' to 'resource mobilisation', 'political process', and 'new social movements'.[13] Edelman argues that, in the 1970s, theorists of new social movements sought to address a number of conceptual conundrums and theoretical blindspots of earlier approaches, in particular the

---

[13] Edelman identifies these paradigm shifts with four major theoretical approaches to understanding collective action in the twentieth century, and draws attention to the conceptual limits of these theories. First, *functionalist frameworks* viewed collective behaviour as irrational mass responses to societal breakdown, but could not explain events such as the counterculture hippy movements of the 1960s that took place amidst almost unprecedented North American affluence and political stability. Second, *rational actor approaches* understood social movements as the sum of participants' strategic individually oriented choices, but could not account for seemingly altruistic decisions taken by 1960s counter-culture students in Europe and North America to 'drop out' of middle-class career trajectories. Third, *traditional Marxist approaches* viewed the bourgeoisie and the proletariat as the central antagonists in capitalist societies, yet it became clear that many of these movements had leaders from middle-class backgrounds and had multi-class constituencies. The fourth approach is that of new social movements (see above).

functionalist and rational actor orientation of these approaches. Edelman identifies Alain Touraine (1974; 1981) as one of the first scholars to theorise the emergence in Europe in the 1970s and 1980s of the 'new' environmentalist, peace and anti-nuclear, women's, gay liberation, minority rights, and student and youth movements (see also Melucci 1989). Since then the list of new movements has grown to include struggles for human rights and democratisation, the rights of indigenous peoples and the needs of the rural landless and urban slum dwellers.

Edelman seeks to make sense of this proliferation of causes by considering the classification of old and new movements. In terms of this conceptual grid, the old social movements were those concerned with old labour or working class struggles in terms of which class was the central social divide, category of analysis, principle of organisation and political issue (1999: 417). The new movements, by contrast, rejected class as the master category and sought to achieve their goals outside of existing institutional channels and party political structures. These new movements were more concerned with questions of cultural struggles over meanings, symbols, collective identities and rights to difference (Alvarez *et al.* 1998; Escobar and Alvarez 1992). Given this cultural turn it is not surprising that these movements have been criticised for being more conservative and reformist than 'older' class-based movements. New social movements (NSMs) have also been criticised for being concerned with questions of cultural recognition, difference and identity in ways that end up reproducing the fragmentation of popular struggles against global capital and its allies.

Implicit in all these analyses is the argument that active citizenship is under siege in this post-political world in which the free market, rapacious consumerism and hyper-individualism reign supreme. This post-political scenario does not completely square up with recent global developments, for instance, the rise of ethno-nationalism from Burundi to the Balkans, and the political fallout in the aftermath of 9/11 – the US invasions of Afghanistan and Iraq, the War on Terror, the rise of militant political Islam, and the subsequent growth of US patriotism and Islamophobia in Europe and North America. Neither does it explain the vibrancy of labour movements in France, South Africa and Brazil, or the spectacular electoral victories of the Left in Latin and South America. In fact, politics seems far from dead and buried in the heartland of Empire and its postcolonial peripheries. As will be demonstrated throughout this book, even in this age of neo-liberalism and global consumerism, collective politics continues to be generated by the contradictions and uneven character of capitalist development in South Africa and beyond. So, while some of these critiques of liberalism may indeed resonate in certain respects with post-apartheid developments – for example in the case of highly individualistic and morally laden biomedical AIDS and tuberculosis treatment and prevention programmes (see Chapters 5 and 6) – the case studies in this book also draw attention to alternative conceptions and outcomes of these forms of self-government and 'responsibilised citizenship'.

The analysis in this book raises questions concerning the universality of these critiques of the post-political era by demonstrating that politics and collective mobilisation are alive and well in post-apartheid South Africa. The analysis draws on case studies of NGOs and social movements that have contributed towards the production of sociality and popular struggles over access to state resources. It also shows how some of these organisations self-consciously draw upon the militant political culture of the anti-apartheid movement while simultaneously introducing new forms of political engagement with the South African state that depart in significant ways from those deployed during the liberation struggle (see Chapter 5). While many commentators on South Africa's transition to democracy predicted the systematic depoliticisation and bureaucratisation of South African society along the lines of Euromodern liberal democracies, the case studies in this book question these universalising and teleological assumptions. The vibrancy and militancy of post-1994 social movements and trade unions, like those in Latin America, suggest that post-apartheid South Africans have not simply morphed into the docile consumer citizens deemed so central to the needs of neoliberal capitalism. There is instead a complex and differentiated transformation afoot in South Africa that defies the simple telos implied in the post-political scenarios sketched by Bauman and others.

Proposition 2: Rights versus culture (and other binaries)

The dichotomies of rights versus culture and modernity versus tradition, have a long history. These binaries recently made a return to political theory on Africa through the work of Mahmood Mamdani (1996) amongst others. In his acclaimed book *Citizen and Subject*, Mamdani draws a neat and categorical line between the liberal individualist citizens of the African city and the ethnic subjects of the countryside. Mamdani's claim that African rural populations continue to consist of ethnic subjects living in 'traditional communities' under the yoke of despotic rulers (traditional authorities) reproduces timeless binaries. Mamdani also argues that the problem with democratisation in post-colonial Africa has been that it left intact the late colonial legacy of indirect rule. Mamdani's analysis – with its urban/rural and citizen/subject dichotomies – does not, however, engage with the complex, hybrid and situated subjectivities of post-colonial citizen-subjects. In its quest for symmetry and conceptual clarity, his account sacrifices the more ambiguous and 'messy' forms of everyday life in the post-colony.

Donors, policy-makers and academics have debated extensively and exhaustively the relationship between liberal individualist notions of citizenship and collectivist conceptions of culture and communal belonging (Cowan, Dembour and Wilson 2001; Mamdani 1996). Numerous ethnographic studies reveal that the conception of the citizen as an atomised and autonomous rights bearing subject is generally at odds with African realities, in terms of which intersubjectivity and interconnectedness are highly valued (Werbner 2002; Nyamnjoh 2002). These studies demonstrate that it is precisely the extreme vulnerability and uncertainty of everyday life in many parts of Africa that demand that postcolonial subjects negotiate their subjection through relationships with others. Clientelism, communitarian forms of citizenship, conviviality and sociality may indeed also be valued precisely for their capacity to hold powerful state actors, traditional leaders and patrons accountable in terms of the delivery of material and social goods (see Chapter 4).

But this does not mean that people in Africa are not open to rights-based approaches when these offer possibilities of access to resources and resolving other social, political, and cultural conflicts. This clearly has implications for social movement and NGO strategies for engaging citizens and states. It suggests that social movements and NGOs, as well as governments and donors, need to recognise that their 'clients' and 'target populations' often live their lives as both citizens and subjects (Nyamnjoh, 2002: 112). What appears to be an autonomous rights-bearing citizen in one setting may, in another context, morph into an 'ethnic' subject invoking indigenous values, traditional beliefs, and forms of sociality and clientelism based on family, clan, neighbourhood and community.

Notwithstanding this political complexity, outmoded modernisation paradigms continue to draw on modern/traditional binaries and timeless conceptions of self-reproducing equilibrium models of African traditional systems, which are regarded as obstacles to progress and development. One implication of this line of thinking is that, with time, Africans will ultimately become just like the liberal citizens of 'the West'. This binary logic implies a citizen versus subject binary, of the sort referred to above. These examples of linear and binary thinking continue to animate contemporary scholarly and policy writing on Africa. This takes place despite a burgeoning literature on 'alternative modernities' (Chakrabarty 1999; Gaonkar 1999),[14] African and Asian modernities (Deutsch, Probst and Schmidt 1999; Ong 1999) and 'alternative democracies' (Paley 2002: 484) that question these binaries of modern and traditional; liberalism and communitarianism; and rights and culture (Cowan, Dembour and Wilson 2001; Ong 1999).

A rejection of these dichotomies can begin to clear the ground for the recognition of the particularities of diverse and situated forms of belonging, rights, citizenship and subjectivity. While scholars still struggle to grasp these hybrid postcolonial realities, activists face them close-up in their everyday encounters with donors, governments and citizens. The NGOs and social movements discussed in this book have developed sophisticated strategies of political engagement that are usually more nuanced than the simplistic binary thinking of many political analysts, donors and media commentators on Africa.

The book will argue that, in postcolonial settings such as South Africa, NGOs and social movement activists increasingly recognise the strategic value of engaging with both liberal 'rights talk' and communal forms of mobilisation. The urban and rural poor also appear to readily acknowledge the need to mobilise collectively in order to stand a chance of realising their individual rights to health care, housing, land, clean water and so on. Indeed, while post-apartheid South Africa has one of the most progressive Constitutions on the planet, for citizens to successfully access these rights usually requires effective and sustained political mobilisation. Even when their organisations have sufficient resources for litigation, activists often recognise that court cases and rights-based claims may need to be supple-

---

[14] Dilip Parameshewar Gaonkar, 1999, 'On Alternative Modernities', *Public Culture*, 11(1): 1–18; Dipesh Chakrabarty, 1999, 'Adda, Calcutta: Dwelling in Modernity', in Dilip Parameshewar Gaonkar (ed.), Alter/ Native Modernities', *Public Culture* 11(1).

mented by grassroots mobilisation. Whereas political theorists regularly juxtapose the citizen and the subject – or rights and culture – as diametrically opposed forms of political engagement, activists and citizens seem to understand the need to straddle rights and ethnic-based discourses. Activists and citizens also do not seem to believe that one form of political engagement (rights) will (or should) eventually replace other forms in a kind of teleological progression.

Proposition 3: Civil society as an elite enclave (but what about the leaks?)

One of the most celebrated and debated concepts to emerge in the so-called post-political era has been civil society. The idea of civil society carries considerable conceptual and symbolic freight in the social sciences and political philosophy, as well as in the streets, the mass media, donor agencies and public spheres. John and Jean Comaroff (1999: 6) write that the term civil society has extraordinary 'transnational appeal as a trope of moral imagining'. Concepts such as democracy, the state and citizenship are equally capable of capturing and generating popular aspirations and moral concerns. While the political meanings and resonance of ideas such as civil society, democracy, rights and citizenship appeared to be relatively clearcut to anti-apartheid activists during the 1980s, their meanings have become increasingly ambiguous in recent years. The post-apartheid period has highlighted the different connotations and competing interpretations of these terms in both popular and elite discourses.

In the West, in the past two decades there has been considerable interest amongst governments and donors in strengthening civil society and creating active citizenship especially in relation to transitions to democracy. In the context of the collapse of the Soviet Union and the fall of the Berlin Wall, as well as popular struggles against apartheid, dictatorships, and military regimes in Africa, Asia and Latin America, civil society came to take on particularly potent significance in the popular imaginary as well as in donor-driven democracy programmes. However, celebrations of civil society and transitions to democracy have, in recent years, given way to cynical assessments, including the circulation of new terms such as low intensity democracy (Gills *et al.* 1993) and democracy lite (Paley 2002: 469). Notwithstanding this disenchantment, the idea of civil society continues to be equated with democratic renewal and this has spurred the proliferation of NGOs. As Steven Sampson[15] noted in an ethnography of a Danish agency involved in democracy programmes in Albania, 'few NGOs meant less democracy, more NGOs meant more democracy' (Sampson 1996: 128, cf. Paley 2002: 482).

Most studies of this democracy industry have been conducted by political scientists interested in questions of procedural democracy and issues relating to formal political institutions, regime transitions, elections and party politics. For instance,

---

[15] Steven Sampson, 1996. 'The social life of projects: importing civil society to Albania', in Hann, C. and Dunn, E. (eds), 1996. Civil Society: *Challenging Western Models*, New York: Routledge, pp. 121–42.

low voter turnout in the United States and Europe spurred numerous studies and democracy programmes concerned with the role of social capital (Putnam 1993), citizen participation, NGOs and voluntary organisations, all viewed as antidotes to these 'democratic deficits'.[16] For many liberal and radical critics alike, civil society organisations continue to be seen as the panacea for promoting active citizenship in contexts of growing voter and civic apathy and depoliticisation.

Notwithstanding this proliferation of studies and programmes, there has been very little ethnographic investigation into what these experiments in strengthening civil society and democracy actually entail. In addition, most accounts of civil society draw on antiquated anthropological and modernisation theory assumptions, which, like bad dreams, keep returning to haunt social scientific thinking. These modernisation narratives imply that Western society has progressed from a 'traditional' to a 'modern' stage of development, and that the non-Western world is still in a state of slow transition towards this Euro-modern future. It is assumed that although non-Western societies remain communitarian in nature they will ultimately come to be characterised by the dominance of universal individualist values of post-Enlightenment Western cultures (Ong 1999: 48). Also implied in this narrative is the idea that modernisation will produce in the non-Western world modern, virtuous citizens along the lines of Euro-modern liberal conceptions of the autonomous rights-bearing subject.

Africa has become a particularly prominent place for donors to exercise this linear and teleological sociological imagination. Civil society organisations and democracy programmes are conceived of as the vehicles for transforming this 'dark continent'. Implied in this liberal modernist narrative is the idea that all human beings will one day become modern consumer citizens.

There have been significant critiques, however, of the cultural and historical assumptions of these Eurocentric ideas (Chatterjee 1993; Comaroff and Comaroff 1999; Hann and Dunn 1996). One critical model of civil society holds that this term refers only to a narrower class of educated elites. Partha Chatterjee (2004: 4) draws on the specific case of India to argue that the term 'civil society' refers to 'a closed association of modern elite groups, sequestered from the wider popular life of the communities, walled up within enclaves of civic freedom and rational law'.[17] These elites constitute the relatively small educated,

---

[16] In an essay entitled *Everyday Democracy*, Tom Bentley, the director of the UK-based democracy think tank *Demos*, seeks to address voter apathy and cynicism by arguing for the rebuilding of UK political culture 'from the bottom up'. He notes that electoral and parliamentary reform and the restructuring of UK political institutions is inadequate without creating opportunities for people to make personal choices in their daily lives in ways that contribute to the common good. See www.demos.co.uk.

[17] Chatterjee (2004: 4) suggests that there is an inherent conflict that 'lies at the heart of modern politics in most of the world ... It is the opposition between the universal ideal of civil nationalism, based on individual freedoms and equal rights irrespective of distinctions of religion, race, language, or culture, and the particular demands of cultural identity, which call for differential treatment of particular groups on grounds of vulnerability or backwardness or historical injustice, or indeed for numerous other reasons.' Chatterjee adds that this opposition is 'symptomatic of the transition that occurred in modern politics in the course of the twentieth century from a conception of democratic politics grounded in the idea of popular sovereignty to one in which democratic politics is shaped by governmentality.'

bourgeois section of the population in Third World countries. The majority of the world's population, Chatterjee argues, belong to the popular classes, what he calls 'political society'. NGOs, social movements and politicians have to navigate between the apparently quite distinct spheres of the state, civil society and the popular classes.

The case studies in this book, however, question the analytic value of both the unquestioning teleological model of civil society as the new democratic common, as well as the more critical analytical separations between the state, civil society and political society. This is especially the case when neat conceptual categories are conflated with complex realities. The borders between these spheres can in fact be extremely porous. For instance, grassroots AIDS activists belonging to TAC became brokers and mediators of biomedical citizenship, rights and popular discourses. They were able to seamlessly straddle these discourses in ways that challenge Chatterjee's conception of civil society as a distinct and sequestered domain of the bourgeois, chattering classes who read newspapers, earn regular salaries, and participate in the liberal democratic public sphere. While there are often divides and tensions between the middle-class leadership and grassroots members of social movements, this does not mean that the latter are completely excluded from the inner sanctum of civil society.

A more useful aspect of Chatterjee's analysis concerns how the popular classes become the 'target populations' of state-driven development and welfare programmes and policies. Chatterjee (2004: 41) writes that they are the subjects of governmentality, which appears to limit their role as agents of mass action and political mobilisation:

> Civil society, then, restricted to a small section of culturally equipped citizens, represents in countries like India the high ground of modernity. So does the constitutional model of the state. But in actual practice, *governmental agencies must descend from that high ground to the terrain of political society* in order to renew their legitimacy as providers of well-being and thereby confront whatever is the current configuration of politically mobilised demands (emphasis added).

This portrait of paternalistic intervention on behalf of needy clients does capture an important aspect of the political dynamics in post-apartheid South Africa. The case studies in this book suggest, however, that 'the popular classes' are not only 'target populations' and 'docile bodies' shaped by, and susceptible to, modern state discourses of development and governmentality; instead they often straddle multiple political discourses and logics in their strategic and situated encounters with the modern state, donor agencies, NGOs, and other sites of power. The chapters on AIDS activism, for example, draw attention to the agency of activists, notwithstanding their intimate engagement with powerful biomedical technologies (e.g., antiretroviral therapy, for example) and state institutions and practices of public health (see Chapters 5, 6 and 7).

Like India, South Africa is a country where the majority of the population seem to stand outside the elite enclaves of Chatterjee's civil society. While acknowledging the value of Chatterjee's analysis, it appears that the borders of this model of civil society are relatively permeable and incorporate members that do not come from the educated middle classes. Similarly, those from the popular classes, as well as members of civil society organisations, sometimes find their way to the upper echelons of the state. The South African liberation struggle, for example, produced thousands of working-class activists who, through their involvement in anti-apartheid activism, were inducted into civil society, and later became significant players in big business and the post-apartheid state. Some, like former deputy president, Jacob Zuma, who had minimal formal schooling, acquired their education and political literacy through decades of involvement in the liberation struggle. Activists such as Zuma were able to take up top positions within the ANC and the post-apartheid state. Similarly, large numbers of rank-and-file trade unionists and township activists made their way into the top echelons of the state and private sector by drawing on struggle networks and political literacies that could be converted into currencies deemed valuable by business and the modern state.

For the majority of South Africans, however, the post-apartheid transition has not provided these kinds of opportunities. With the arrival of democracy in 1994, many highly effective grassroots activists were unable to convert their political skills and credentials into the forms of cultural capital required by the new bureaucratic state. Jobless growth and structural unemployment have created barriers to upward mobility and participation in middle-class civil society. This does not mean, however, that the excluded masses are living in some pre-modern political and cultural backwater. Moreover, millions of black working-class South Africans are highly literate in the language of rights, equality, citizenship and social justice. Members of civil society organisations, as well as ordinary citizens, seem particularly adept at straddling elite and popular discourses and deploying the state's discourses of rights, citizenship and development. However, access to these political literacies is no guarantee of access to jobs or full membership of the inner circle of middle-class civil society.

The conceptual opposition posited by Chatterjee (2004) – between the state, civil society and political society – collapses under the weight of the everyday social realities of those living in the margins of the South African state and the formal economy, that is the majority of South Africa's population. For most South Africans, claiming rights is not necessarily incompatible with claiming communitarian identities and cultural and group rights. Both of these purportedly antagonistic and oppositional political logics can be asserted by the same actors simultaneously, or deployed separately depending on the specific contexts and audiences.

Rather than subscribing to the binary logics and neat analytic categories of Mamdani's and Chatterjee's political theories, this book argues that most people in South Africa act as both citizens and subjects, and they strategically and situationally engage with 'rights talk' and the political discourses of liberal democracy. In other words, they do not seem to be straightjacketed into the categories and political spheres, like 'civil society', that analysts seek to impose upon them. Citizens and subjects in many parts of the global South straddle the continuum of political discourses that stretch between the poles of 'liberal rights' and 'communitarian cultures'.

The central argument in this book is that in post-apartheid South Africa, innovative NGO-social movement strategic partnerships – for instance, between People's

Dialogue (PD) and the SA Homeless People's Federation (SAHPF) (Chapter 4), and *Médecins Sans Frontières* (MSF) and TAC (Chapter 5) – have played a central role in mediating between state-centric rights discourses and popular politics. They have also blurred the borders between the domains of civil society and the popular classes, thereby complicating Chatterjee's model. The case studies draw attention to the highly improvisational and situational character of these experimental forms of NGO-social movement mobilisation in the margins of the state and global capitalism.

Rights and revolution during apartheid

Recent South African history can be narrated as an epic revolutionary struggle against an oppressive apartheid regime. It can also be framed as a liberal modernist struggle for democratic rights that began in 1912 with the formation of the ANC and came to fruition in 1994 with the inauguration of President Nelson Mandela as president of the new democratic South Africa. Events such as the Treason Trial of 1956, the Rivonia Trial in 1963, when Mandela and the top leadership of the ANC were sentenced to long-term imprisonment on Robben Island, the Sharpeville massacre of 1961, and the Soweto Uprising of 1976 were key moments in this long march to freedom.

This historical account usually focuses on the vanguard role of modernising nationalist elites: Nelson Mandela, Oliver Tambo, Walter Sisulu, Govan Mbeki, Joe Slovo, Chris Hani and numerous other icons of the liberation struggle. These modernising nationalists challenged the legitimacy of traditional leaders who, together with the apartheid state, propped up the ethnic 'homelands' and nation states. They dismissed traditional leaders as backward and anti-democratic collaborators in the indirect rule policies of the colonial and apartheid regimes. They also rejected the legitimacy of the homelands – Transkei, Ciskei, Bophuthatswana, Venda, Qwaqwa, Lebowa, Gazankulu, KwaNdebele, and KwaZulu.[18] From the perspective of the ANC's revolutionary leadership, homelands and traditional leadership had to be systematically dismantled. These separate development policies created the conditions for mass resistance to apartheid's urban influx control measures and ultimately led to the massive growth of shantytowns in South Africa's cities.[19] They also swelled the ranks of anti-apartheid civic organisations and the liberation movements.

---

[18] The homelands were overcrowded and impoverished rural reserves that functioned as 'ethnic' dumping grounds for 'surplus' and 'redundant' black South Africans whose labour was not required in 'white' South Africa. Hundreds of thousands of Black South Africans who were officially classified as Zulu, Xhosa, Tsonga, Venda, Tswana, Sotho, Ndebele, and Pedi, were forcibly removed from these 'white areas' (referred to as 'black spots'), which included all the major cities and about 80 per cent of viable agricultural land. As 'citizens' of these ethnic homelands and nation-states, they were stripped of their South African citizenship. They were relocated to underdeveloped homelands where they were told they could exercise their political, cultural and economic rights.

[19] In response to these Separate Development policies, progressive intellectuals and anti-apartheid activists identified ethnic-based politics and participation in Tribal Authorities structures as overt collusion with apartheid 'divide and rule' strategies. It was also not surprising that anti-apartheid intellectuals and activists drew on Marxism and Steve Biko's Black Consciousness Movement to challenge ethnicity and 'tribalism' as forms of 'false consciousness'.

During the height of apartheid in the 1970s, Marxist intellectuals within the liberation movements developed powerful critiques of liberal political theorists who argued that apartheid was simply an irrational and backward political system whose racial laws were an obstacle to the emergence of modern, free market capitalism. Marxists such as Harold Wolpe challenged this view by arguing that the apartheid state system was a specific form of racial capitalism that could only be transformed through radical transformations in the relations of production. From this perspective, apartheid's racial policies underpinned forms of labour control and exploitation that had to be systematically dismantled; it was insufficient to simply get rid of racially based legislation. Rights and legal reform alone would be inadequate. What was actually required was the revolutionary seizure of state power and the nationalisation of key assets such as land and the mines.

By the mid-1990s, however, the new ANC-led government appeared to abandon theories of socialist revolution for liberal democracy and IMF-friendly neo-liberal macro-economic policies.[20] Whereas the Left within the ANC subscribed to a 'two-stage theory' in terms of which national liberation would be followed by socialist transformation, by the early 1990s it had become clear that the second stage had been indefinitely stalled.

Throughout the mid-1980s a proliferation of mostly urban-based civic, labour, and community-based organisations challenged the apartheid state using the liberal language of rights, citizenship and democracy alongside the radical rhetoric of revolutionary struggle and national liberation. These anti-apartheid organisations, which were affiliated to the United Democratic Front (UDF), also rejected the Bantustan system and instead called for the creation of a unitary, non-racial democratic nation-state. The UDF comprised a broad coalition of hundreds of organisations and came to be seen as the 'internal wing' of the ANC.[21] The ANC and UDF, together with a range of other anti-apartheid organisations, ultimately brought the repressive apartheid state to its knees. In 1990, former president F.W. de Klerk began the negotiation process by announcing the release of Nelson Mandela and unbanning the liberation movements. This brief historical sketch of the road to democracy shows how liberal, socialist and 'ethnic' political discourses have always been intertwined in political life in South Africa. Rhetorics and strategies may have changed with new circumstances and 'enemies', but it has always been complex and situational. It is precisely the hybrid and improvisional quality of politics in South Africa that is explored in the case studies that follow.

---

[20] The 1990s also witnessed post-modernist and post-structural theory and cultural studies replacing Marxism in the curricula of most South African universities. Studies of new social movements, 'civil society' and 'rights' were deemed useful for understanding South African political realities. Since the demise of Marxism, however, there has been very little systematic theorisation of the South African state. While there have been some attempts to analyse the South African state as a standardised neo-liberal state, these have tended to be formulaic and have often failed to take cognisance of the fact that the South African state's social spending budget is massive by any standards. Neither have such analyses fully addressed the competing ideological and political tendencies within the Tripartite Alliance of the ANC, South African Communist Party (SACP) and the Congress of South African Trade Unions (COSATU).

[21] There were also militant political movements such as the Pan–Africanist Congress (PAC), the Azanian People's Organisation (AZAPO), the New Unity Movement and Qibla.

Strategic partnerships: NGOs and social movements after apartheid

While the legacies of the political culture of the anti-apartheid struggle remain, a plethora of new community-based organisations and social movements have emerged since the mid-1990s that depart from the more militant and revolutionary political styles, objectives and modes of mobilisation of the apartheid era. Most post-apartheid social movements and NGOs have adopted pragmatic strategies to access donor funds and state resources. Meanwhile, the ANC has transformed itself from a revolutionary liberation movement into a political party, a bureaucratic machine and a corporate state structure. These seismic shifts have resulted in surprising outcomes. For example, while there was considerable popular resistance to the Bantustan system in the 1980s, during the 1990s there were efforts by the ANC government to rehabilitate former Bantustan traditional leaders and ethnic political entrepreneurs. Apartheid-era ethnic politics transmogrified into rights-based community claims for access to land, culture and language. The Truth & Reconciliation Commission (TRC) and the Land Restitution processes also drew on rights-based approaches to redress the apartheid past.

Alongside this dramatic shift from revolution to rights has been the emergence of new forms of ethnogenesis in terms of which identity and community are reconstituted through cultural and intellectual property rights. These new forms of 'ethnic' mobilisation sometimes involve lucrative business deals. For example, following their successful land claim in 1999, the ≠khomani San's lawyer Roger Chennels, together with the South African San Institute (SASI), entered into negotiations to sell San crafts to dollar-laden tourists who shop at the upmarket stores at South Africa's international airports. Another San success came out of negotiations over the sale of indigenous San knowledge concerning the use of the *Hoodia gordonii* plant to a global pharmaceutical company interested in marketing the plant as a natural appetite suppressant and weight loss product (see Chapter 3). While the San land claim itself has not generated significant income, Chennels' negotiation of the San crafts and *Hoodia* deals certainly has.

These forms of commodification of culture and indigenous knowledge can be aptly described as *Ethnicity Inc.*(see Comaroff & Comaroff forthcoming). Another example of this phenomenon is the case of the Bafokeng Kingdom of North West Province[22] which in 1999, won a 10-year legal battle for royalty payments from Impala Platinum Holdings (Implats). These payments, which were calculated on the basis that Implats had mined platinum on Bafokeng land since the 1960s, amounted to an estimated R827 million at the end of the 2002 financial year. The Bafokeng have used these massive deposits of platinum, the largest outside of Russia, to reproduce 'tribal' traditions and build modern infrastructure including schools, clinics, hospitals, sports and recreation facilities and a major Science and Technology Academy.

---

[22] The 'Bafokeng nation' extends over 70,000 hectares and is sub-divided into 72 traditional *dikgoro* (wards), each of which is regulated by a hereditary *dikgosana* (headman) and *mmadikgosana* (headman's wife). An anthropologist, Susan Cook, has done extensive work on the Bafokeng Kingdom.

It would seem that access to these resources – indigenous knowledge and platinum deposits – have facilitated the 'reinvention' of these indigenous communities. These processes reveal new ways in which NGO lawyers are assisting communities to draw on intellectual and cultural property rights in order to access resources that can then be used both to reconstitute collective identity and hasten modern forms of socio-economic development. The case studies summarised below demonstrate that rights-based struggles such as those forged by the San, do not merely produce post-political conditions of liberal individualism, as some critics suggest. Neither are these rights-based approaches necessarily incompatible with more conventional forms of collective action and cultural reproduction.

While a fledgling indigenous rights movement was emerging in rural Namaqualand in the 1990s, a number of militant social movements were flexing their muscles throughout South Africa. These included anti-globalisation and popular Left movements that challenged what they perceived to be the neo-liberal capitulation of the ANC government. Left intellectuals within these movements, including those based at the Centre for Civil Society in Durban, regarded the transition from apartheid as a form of 'elite pacting' that killed the socialist revolution and replaced it with a capital-friendly, neo-liberal democracy (Bond 2000; Marais 1998).[23] They blamed the ANC government's macro-economic policies for contributing to jobless growth, the privatisation of state assets, and a downsized neo-liberal state. The shortcomings of the post-apartheid state in the realm of socio-economic transformation, jobs, housing and social services have allowed civil society organisations, including NGOs and new social movements, to step into the breach.

Since 1994 the following social movements have come into existence: the South African Homeless People's Federation (1994), the Treatment Action Campaign (1998), the Concerned Citizens Forum (1999), the Anti-Eviction Campaign, the Anti-Privatisation Forum, the Soweto Electricity Crisis Committee (2000), the Landless Peoples Movement, the Coalition of South Africans for the Basic Income Grant (2001), Abahlali base Mjondolo (The Durban Shack Dwellers' Movement 2005). The formation of these movements can be seen as civil society responses to the perceived failures of the post-apartheid state to address issues of HIV/AIDS, land redistribution, job creation, housing, poverty, etc.

Although South Africa has a vibrant civil society comprising hundreds of NGOs and civil society organisations, this book focuses specifically on three NGO-social

[23]   See Bond, 2000. *Elite Transition: From Apartheid to Neoliberalism in South Africa*. London: Pluto Press. Marais, H. 1998. *South Africa: Limits to Change: The Political Economy of Transformation*. London: Zed Books. Left critics such as Patrick Bond and Hein Marais argue that the ANC ruling elite has abandoned the Freedom Charter's brand of socialism and replaced its vision of the interventionist Development State with that of the downsized neo-liberal state. It is these macro-economic policies, Left critics argue, that have led to jobless growth, major cutbacks in government social expenditure, cost recovery measures and privatisation of services such as water, electricity and transport, and the cutting off of essential services for those in arrears. From this perspective, the ANC's current macro-economic policies are perceived to be exacerbating historically produced inequalities. This failure to improve the conditions of the bottom 50 per cent of the population has occurred despite moderate rates of inflation, a growing economy, 1.3 million extra telephone connections, clean water for an extra 9 million people, electricity for 1.5 million more, and thousands of new classrooms and clinics. Critics conclude that despite the benefits of a progressive Constitution and an improvement in the delivery of services, South Africa continues to have one of the most unequal income distribution curves in the world.

movement partnerships that have been involved in collective mobilisation by establishing an indigenous peoples movement, a transnational urban poor movement, and a globally connected AIDS activist movement. While there are distinct bodies of literature on NGOs and social movements, this book is one of very few that investigates the specific dynamics of NGO-social movement partnerships. It is significant to note that many of the most successful forms of political mobilisation after apartheid have come in the form of these NGO-social movement partnerships. This book explores the conceptual and empirical dimensions of these partnerships and shows how they are responsible for introducing news forms of rights-based political mobilisation. It will also be argued that these partnerships have contributed towards expanding conventional conceptions of civil society, rights and citizenship.

In all of the cases discussed in the book, the grassroots participants in these social movements were from marginalised communities, and these experiments in rights-claiming and collective mobilisation took place after apartheid. The Nama (Khoi) and San communities in the Northern Cape Province, the Xhosa-speaking women belonging to the SAHPF, and the predominantly black working class AIDS activists of TAC, have also all had the common experience of living on the margins of South Africa's modern capitalist economy. A central problem for these NGO–social movement partnerships has been to create conditions of social belonging and solidarity for people living at the margins of the state and the formal economy. This is particularly difficult given the ways in which poverty tends to reproduce conditions of social fragmentation, anomie and isolation. How then do NGOs and social movements go about deploying rights-based approaches and producing new forms of solidarity and sociality amongst such marginalised populations? How are such solidarities and forms of collective mobilisation produced in post-revolutionary settings such as South Africa, where neo-liberal capitalism and rampant consumer culture appear to be the only games in town?

NGOs, social movements, the state and beyond

Notwithstanding the structural constraints and 'limits of liberation' (Robins 2005) that have been identified by Left critics of neo-liberalism, South Africa has a relatively 'Big State' that includes a progressive Constitution that enshrines socio-economic rights, as well as a public sector with considerable resources at its disposal, including significant military and security capacity and social welfare, housing, land redistribution and public health programmes.[24] Millions of marginalised citizens perceive engagement with the post-apartheid state and its programmes as an important element in their multi-stranded and multi-sited survival strategies. These fluid and dispersed multi-sited livelihood strategies are deployed in a hostile economic environment where long-term employment is

[24] It is also evident that the South African state remains a key player for NGOs, social movements and millions of citizens. Given the wealth, size and reach of the South Africa state, it is not surprising that civil society actors and citizens take the State seriously. This is not the kind of despotic and authoritarian state caricatured in much contemporary scholarly and media commentary on Africa. Neither is it the classical right-sized neo-liberal state that is routinely denounced by some Left critics.

increasingly difficult to find and the casualisation of labour and informalisation of the economy look likely to stay. Yet, pensions and welfare and disability grants, along with housing subsidies, continue to feature centrally in the lives of millions of poor people. These conditions make it difficult if not impossible for the South African state and civil society actors to totally capture the loyalties of its citizens. At the same time, the South African state is sufficiently well resourced to ensure that its citizens cannot afford to completely circumvent or ignore it.

As a consequence, the urban and rural poor in South Africa, as well as elsewhere in the developing world, commit enormous resources and energy to ensuring the social reproduction of kinship, clientship, clan, and neighbourhood ties and networks. Given prevailing conditions of jobless growth and structural unemployment, it is not surprising that these social bonds are seldom sacrificed for the elusive dream of 'suburban bliss' with its normative model of the nuclear family, private property and individual, bourgeois subjectivity.

It is in this context – of a 'big', but distrusted state, and a welter of other possible networks and strategies for social reproduction – that the NGO has flourished in post-apartheid South Africa. Many see this growth as an index of the health of its democracy. Certainly, NGOs are often associated with the virtuous values of civil society, development, democracy and accountability. The mainstream NGO literature tends to portray NGOs as autonomous, participatory and accountable. These days, however, such descriptions of NGOs are also routinely deconstructed as 'NGO myths'. Over the past few years, it has become increasingly common to hear that NGOs have become the handmaidens of neoliberalism and global capital (Hardt and Negri 2000; Kamat 2003, 2005; Petras and Veltmeyer 2001).

Critics claim that NGOs have lost their critical edge as they have come increasingly under pressure to manage their programmes on a profitable basis, with state subsidies being cut and soft loans and grants for development programmes being minimised by the IMF and World Bank via Structural Adjustment Programmes (SAPs) (Kamat 2005:152). Some have argued that the term 'franchise state' accurately describes the new relations between NGOs and the state in neoliberal contexts wherein NGOs subcontract the management and administration of essential services from the state (see Alvarez 1998; Petras 1997). Similarly, Sonia Alvarez (1998: 152) argues that there has been a transformation of radical feminist movements in Latin America, what she calls the 'NGOisation of feminism,' that has resulted in women's issues being professionally managed in ways that are similar to state institutions. NGOs are also routinely challenged for introducing processes of individualisation and depoliticisation that undermine the possibility of collective mobilisation and promote the interests of the state and neoliberal capital. For instance, Sangeeta Kamat (2005: 148) argues that NGOs are often responsible for 'normalising' a form of rights-based politics that is only acceptable within a narrowly circumscribed liberal democratic framework.

South African NGOs have faced similar accusations and criticisms. For instance, NGOs such as *Médecins Sans Frontières* (MSF) and TAC activists are routinely accused by AIDS dissidents, including those in the ruling party, of being 'salespersons' and fronts of the global pharmaceutical industry. Similarly, the South African government and President Mbeki's spokespersons have labelled anti-globalisation NGOs and social movements as 'ultra-Leftist' groupings with unpatriotic agendas and shadowy foreign affiliations.

These critiques of NGOs are also emerging in a context of growing donor interest in democracy programmes that seek to promote community participation, state accountability, citizen empowerment, and social capital. Left critics argue that these Western donor interests dovetail neatly with 'anti-statist' neo-liberal programmes of structural adjustment. These donor interests are also often seen to be part of strategies by the World Bank, IMF, WTO and other global financial institutions to impose economic liberalisation policies and the downsizing of states, especially those in the Third World.

A particularly harsh critique of NGOs can be found in Michael Hardt and Antonio Negri's (2000) *Empire*. Hardt and Negri state that 'moral interventions' by NGOs may be more significant than military intervention in shoring up the sovereignty of the new political order of globalisation that they refer to as *Empire*.[25] For Hardt and Negri, NGOs are especially well placed to do this work of moral intervention 'precisely because they are not run directly by governments, [and] are assumed to act on the basis of ethical or moral imperatives' (ibid: 35–6). Hardt and Negri regard humanitarian NGOs such as Amnesty International, Oxfam, and MSF as 'some of the most powerful pacific weapons of the new world order – the charitable campaigns and the mendicant orders of Empire' (ibid: 36). These NGOs, they argue, 'conduct "just war" without arms, without violence, without borders' (ibid). Comparing them to Dominican and Jesuit missionaries of earlier incarnations of Empire, Hardt and Negri claim that these organisations 'strive to identify universal needs and defend human rights' while simultaneously clearing the moral ground for military intervention and internationally sanctioned police action.

These sweeping critiques of NGOs as the handmaidens of Empire can in turn be criticised for failing to acknowledge the heterogeneous character of NGOs and development agencies. Given the differentiation in the forms, functions and relationships of NGOs, how can Hardt and Negri legitimately label all NGOs in the Third World as mere servants of the neo-liberal project of global capital?[26] How can such a heterogeneous category share common ideological and political agendas? These critiques also make no reference to the complex and situational ways in which 'beneficiaries' engage with NGOs. Agency, subjectivity and unintended outcomes are alien concepts in their searing criticisms of NGOs and 'development'.

Like the interventions of Christian missionaries before them, the ultimate

---

[25] For Hardt and Negri, Empire represents a new political order of globalisation that ushers in a universal order that accepts no boundaries or limits. This newly emerging Empire is contrasted with the imperialism of European dominance and capitalist expansion of earlier epochs. Today's global Empire assimilates elements of US constitutionalism in ways that undermine the foundations of the nation, ethnicity, race and peoples by multiplying the instances of contact and hybridisation. In this way it transforms sovereignty into a system of diffuse national and supranational institutions.

[26] Hardt and Negri isolate a specific subset of NGOs, i.e., humanitarian organisations that include human rights organisations (such as Amnesty International and Americas Watch), peace groups, and the medical and famine relief agencies (such as Oxfam and *Médecins sans Frontières*) (313). Hardt and Negri's interest in these particular agencies arises from their observation that 'the activities of these NGOs coincide with the workings of Empire "beyond politics," on the terrain of biopower, meeting the needs of life itself' (313–14).

outcomes of NGO projects are often unanticipated and counter-intuitive. Early twentieth-century missionaries, for example, could not have anticipated that missionary education would later be seen as the catalyst for the emergence of a critical black consciousness that contributed towards the ANC's revolutionary struggle against apartheid; similarly, today's donors and NGOs cannot be entirely sure what their interventions will end up looking like. Regardless of the mission statements and ideological commitments of their donor supporters in Europe and North America, NGOs in developing countries usually recognise that they need to 'indigenise' their projects in ways that resonate with the needs and popular aspirations in the particular settings within which they work. The pragmatic imperatives of having to intervene and mobilise at local, national, regional and global levels require sophisticated localised strategies and discursive framings. None of this complexity and agency is evident in Negri and Hardt's totalising critiques of NGOs. Neither do they acknowledge the efficacy of the mobilisation strategies of NGO–social movement partnerships that successfully leverage access to state resources for hyper-marginalised populations.

In sum, there are two schools of thought on NGOs. The first school views them as benevolent agencies that provide solutions to political and humanitarian crises that states and markets cannot and/or are unwilling to address – poverty, famine, torture, starvation, massacre, imprisonment and social justice, for example. In contrast, critics regard NGOs as the ideological conduits of neo-liberal capital (Petras and Veltmeyer 2001; Petras 1987). For example, James Petras argues that 'while global capital attacks the powers of the nation-state from above, NGOs attack "from below", presenting the community face of neo-liberalism'. Both schools of thought seem to agree, however, that the growth of global capital has contributed towards a reduction in the autonomy and reach of the state, and created opportunities for the dramatic expansion of an international civil society. The retreat of the neo-liberal state has also created the conditions for the emergence of global civic action that presents alternative discourses of development and democraticisation (see Escobar and Alvarez 1992; Escobar 1995).

There has not only been a massive explosion in the numbers of NGOs but also a dramatic emergence of new functions and organisational linkages. William Fisher (1997: 441) notes, for example, that NGOs have 'forged complex and wide-ranging formal and informal linkages with one another, with government agencies, with social movements, with international development agencies, with individual INGOs (international NGOs), and with transnational issue networks'. But do these linkages constitute the constellation of networks that Hardt and Negri describe as 'Empire'? Are NGOs the conduits of global capital and processes of individualisation, depoliticisation and neo-liberalism? Have the anti-apartheid NGOs and social movements of the liberation struggle in South Africa merely transmogrified into the ideological instruments of Empire?

The case studies in this book will show that while NGOs and social movements are indeed often the mediators of liberal modernist ideas and practices relating to rights and citizenship, this need not be at the behest of global capital or at the expense of popular forms of collective mobilisation. Furthermore, adopting rights-based approaches does not automatically transform 'beneficiaries' into 'lone citizens' whose consciousness is completely colonised by liberal individualist conceptions of citizenship. The roles and outcomes of NGO interventions are considerably more complicated. The case studies in this book draw attention to these partnerships' capacity to straddle both rights-based politics and collective forms of mobilisation.

Chapter summaries

The chapters in this book were mostly written in the decade after South Africa's first democratic elections in 1994. I had returned to South Africa in 1993 after having studied anthropology at Columbia University in New York and completed my doctoral thesis on land redistribution in Zimbabwe. Soon after my return to South Africa, I turned my ethnographic attention to some striking new developments in post-apartheid political life. I became increasingly interested in the complex ways in which NGOs and civic activists in Namaqualand's Reserves in the Northern Cape Province were making connections between the ANC's ideology of 'non-racialism' and national liberation and new forms of indigenous identity politics, in this case Nama (Khoi) identity (see Chapter 2). By focusing on indigenous land rights, these NGOs and community activists also came into increasing contact with globally connected indigenous rights movements in Australia, New Zealand, North America and elsewhere.

This politics of indigenous identity looked very different to anti-apartheid modes of mass mobilisation with their emphasis on class, race and nation. As an anthropology student at the University of Cape Town (UCT) in the early 1980s, I had been drawn to Marxism's ability to make sense of the political implications of the underlying economic structures of apartheid, or what the Left then referred to as a specific form of racial capitalism. According to this economistic logic, matters relating to culture, identity and religion were simply superstructural reflections of the underlying economic base. My BA Honours ethnographic research had focused on the social and economic impact of the forced removal of hundreds of thousands of ex-farm workers and their families from Orange Free State commercial farms to the overcrowded and impoverished South Sotho ethnic 'homeland' of Qwaqwa. These removals of labour rendered 'surplus' by the increasing mechanisation on white commercial farms, highlighted the devastating consequences of apartheid's Bantustan policies. At the time, these developments seemed to reveal the brutal machinations of an unbridled and rapacious species of racial capitalism.

A decade later, studying indigenous identity in the Northern Cape in the mid-1990s entailed a major intellectual shift. Studying identity rather than the effects of capitalism reflected the seismic political and intellectual shifts of the period: the collapse of state socialism in Eastern Europe, the decline of Marxism in the academy, the 'cultural turn' and growing influence of post-structuralism and post-modernism. It was within this dramatically changed political and intellectual milieu, as well as South Africa's own particular post-apartheid twists and turns, that identity politics became central to my work. However, the social organisation and strategies of identity politics after apartheid were strikingly different to identity politics in the North.

This difference was reflected in the rise of new social movements that deployed both rights-based activism and popular forms of collective mobilisation that were similar, in many respects, to the political culture of the anti-apartheid struggle. It was the emergence of new transnational social movements that captured my attention, and ultimately led me to focus on globally connected forms of land, housing and AIDS activism, or what has come to be understood as 'globalisation from below' (see Chapters 3, 4 and 5). The focus on AIDS activism was perhaps to be expected, given concerns about a devastating pandemic that had, by 2008, resulted in the infection of 6 million South Africans (see Chapters 5, 6 and 7).

Chapter 2 discusses how, in the late 1980s, South Africa witnessed the first rumblings of an indigenous rights movement. This took place when 'Coloured' communal farmers in the North Cape Province 'Coloured Reserves' reclaimed their Nama identity in the course of their struggles against apartheid state initiatives aimed at privatising the commons. These communities, together with their NGO allies, drew on rights-based legal discourses to buttress their claims that they were the living embodiment of indigenous Nama culture in terms of which private property had no place or precedent. This 'ethnic revitalisation' movement contributed towards wider attempts to reclaim Khoi and San culture, history and identity after apartheid. In fact, it signalled the beginnings of a South African indigenous rights movement. This case study supports the central argument of the book by showing how activists and marginalised communities straddled the rights versus culture divide.

Chapter 3 takes up a similar theme. This case demonstrates how Afrikaans-speaking ex-farm workers in the North Cape Province, together with their lawyers and NGO allies, successfully used the ANC government's Land Restitution Act to win a land claim that created the conditions for them to reconstitute themselves as 'bushmen' hunter-gatherers. The case focuses on the cultural politics of the ≠khomani San land claim in the Kalahari in the Northern Cape Province. Like the Namaqualand case, the San land claim contributed towards the growth in South Africa of a globally connected indigenous peoples movement. It also encouraged South African anthropologists to critically engage with anthropological and cultural studies debates on 'the invention of tradition' (Hobsbawm and Ranger 1983), 'staged ethnicity' (Boonzaier and Sharp 1994; Robins 1997), 'hybridity' (Appiah 1992; Bhabha 1990; Gilroy 1993) and 'strategic essentialism' (Spivak 1988). The case study illustrates the tensions and contradictions that arise when donors and NGOs deploy essentialist indigenous discourses of 'traditional bushmen' alongside liberal individualist rights talk. It also draws attention to the creative agency and hybrid repertoire of strategies used by 'bushmen' citizen-subjects who are constituted as beneficiaries of nation-state and global donor and NGO programmes and projects.

Chapter 4 focuses on the activist ideology, practices and networks of the People's

Dialogue (PD), an NGO that established a strategic partnership with the South African Homeless People's Federation (SAHPF), a transnational urban poor movement. The case study draws attention to the disjuncture between the official ideology of the Slum Dwellers International (SDI), to which both PD and the SAHPF are affiliated, and the everyday ideas and practices of the rank-and-file members of the SAHPF. It shows how the horizontal, non-party-political, non-hierarchical, democratic ideology of PD and SDI came to clash with the ANC patronage networks and leadership cliques that developed amongst the grassroots housing activists in the townships. Whereas SDI and PD were interested in promoting horizontal forms of social capital and deep democracy, a small group of veteran housing activist leaders used their connections to the ANC and NGO leadership in order to entrench hierarchies and amass personal and material power. The case study focuses on the complex forms of mobilisation deployed by PD and SAHPF activists to leverage access to donor funding and state housing subsidies. It also interrogates the SDI concept of deep democracy and highlights tensions between rights-based approaches to 'development' and locally embedded political cultures of patronage, hierarchy and authority. The case study ultimately begs the question: how deep is deep democracy and how grassroots is 'grassroots globalisation' (see Appadurai 2001)?

Chapter 5 also takes up this theme of grassroots globalisation in its investigation of AIDS activism and the politics of science, citizenship and cultural nationalism in South Africa. It shows how MSF and TAC created an extraordinarily effective NGO–social movement partnership that resembled, in many respects, the SDI model of 'globalisation from below' (see Chapter 4, and Appadurai 2001, Falk 1993).[27] It also shows how an NGO–social movement partnership was able to effectively deploy both rights-based approaches and community-based, but globally connected, forms of social mobilisation. TAC captured the imagination of AIDS activists, journalists and supporters throughout the world in their David and Goliath legal battles for anti-AIDS drugs. Formed in Cape Town in 1998, TAC emerged as a globally connected social movement that successfully used the courts, the media, and social mobilisation in the townships, to persuade global pharmaceutical giants and the South African government to put measures in place for the provision of AIDS treatment.

Chapter 6 follows on from the previous chapter by focusing on the illness narratives and treatment testimonies of former MSF and TAC activists. It investigates how an emerging moral politics of AIDS activism in South Africa has contributed towards new forms of 'caring for the self' and self-fashioning that Vihn-Kim Nguyen calls 'therapeutic citizenship' (Nguyen 2005). The chapter investigates the relationship between the rights-based approach of TAC, and the social movement's processes of building collective identity and belonging. It argues that people living with AIDS in South Africa and elsewhere are not simply autonomous rights-bear-

---

[27] Falk (1993) first introduced the concept of 'globalization-from-below' to refer to a global civil society in ways that explicitly challenged elite and corporate-led 'globalization-from-above'. See Falk, R. 1993. 'The Making of Global Citizenship' in Childs, J.B., Brecher, J. and Cutler, J. (eds) *Global Visions: Beyond the New World Order*, Boston, MA: South End, pp. 39–50.

ing citizens seeking state health and social welfare resources; they are also active members of a strong social movement. This chapter argues that it was precisely the extremity of 'near death' experiences of full-blown AIDS, and the profound stigma and 'social death' associated with the later stages of the disease, that produced the conditions for AIDS survivors' commitment to 'new life', 'responsibilised citizenship' and social activism. These profound changes at the level of subjectivity and identity produced forms of 'responsibilised citizenship' that were simultaneously highly individualised and socially and politically active. They emerged from near death into a new life both as objects of individualising biomedical interventions as well as the subjects of a collective social movement.

Chapter 7 focuses on post-apartheid masculinities in relation to, firstly, the sexual politics that surrounded the 2006 rape trial of the former Deputy President Jacob Zuma, and second the establishment of Khululeka, a community-based HIV men's support group in Gugulethu, Cape Town. These two cases, it will be argued, reveal new forms of sexual politics that highlight competing conceptions of rights, morality, religion, culture and political leadership. They also reveal the tensions between liberal sexual rights and patriarchal sexual cultures, for instance, and the gap between South Africa's progressive constitution and the everyday realities of gender and sexual inequality. Like the other chapters, this case study shows how NGOs and community-based activists seek to navigate their way through this contested terrain.

2

Activist Mediations of 'Rights' & Indigenous Identity
Land Struggles, NGOs & Indigenous Rights in Namaqualand

I am an African.

I owe my being to the hills and the valleys, the mountains and the glades, the rivers, the deserts, the trees, the flowers, the seas and the ever-changing seasons that define the face of our native land.

I owe my being to the Khoi and the San whose desolate souls haunt the great expanses of the beautiful Cape – they who fell victim to the most merciless genocide our native land has ever seen, they who were the first to lose their lives in the struggle to defend our freedom and dependence and they who, as a people, perished in the result.

Today, as a country, we keep an audible silence about these ancestors of the generations that live, fearful to admit the horror of a former deed, seeking to obliterate from our memories a cruel occurrence which, in its remembering, should teach us not and never to be inhuman again.

(Statement of Deputy President Thabo Mbeki, on behalf of the African National Congress on the occasion of the adoption by the Constitutional Assembly of the Republic of South Africa Constitutional Bill 1996; Cape Town, 8 May 1996)

During the apartheid period, it was widely believed that indigenous Nama and San people had become 'extinct' or else assimilated into the 'Coloured' population. In fact, in 1996 Deputy President Mbeki made a similar claim about the Khoi and the San having perished in 'the most merciless genocide our native land has ever seen'. Yet, in the mid-1990s, Nama and San people were becoming increasingly visible in the public sphere as they turned to the courts to reclaim land from which they were evicted under apartheid. In 1998 the 4000-strong indigenous Nama (Khoi) community in the Richtersveld Reserves of Namaqualand in the Northern Cape Province began a legal battle to reclaim land from which they were removed in 1927. In 2006, following lengthy litigation, they eventually won the case and were awarded financial compensation. Similarly, in 1999, the ≠khomani San won back land from which they were evicted by the apartheid state (see Chapter 3). In both cases, lawyers and NGO field workers from the Legal Resources Centre (LRC), the Surplus Peoples Project (SPP) and the South African San Institute (SASI) played a central role in both the litigation and contributing towards the emergence of an indigenous rights movement in South Africa. The LRC and SPP had a long history of assisting communities against apartheid evictions and forced removals. They had developed effective methods for combining litigation with mass mobilisation. These land restitution cases on behalf of indigenous people in the Northern Cape Province revealed that methods of anti-apartheid legal activism were being carried over into the post-apartheid period. These restitution cases played a significant role in revitalising and legitimising the reclaiming of Nama and ≠khomani San identity in the Northern Cape Province.

The first section of the chapter focuses on the early beginnings of an indigenous rights movement in Namaqualand's' 'Coloured Reserves,' as well as the responses of South African anthropologists to these post-apartheid developments. In this section I argue that South African anthropologists have tended to misread the political logics and forms of 'strategic essentialism'[1] deployed by indigenous rights activists in their attempts to straddle discourses on rights and culture. I also critique anthropologists who have used notions of 'invented tradition' (Hobsbawm and Ranger 1983) and 'staged ethnicity' (Boonzaier and Sharp 1994) to understand the emergence of indigenous identity politics in the Northern Cape Province in the 1990s. The second section focuses specifically on the complex ways in which community activists sought to translate and mediate 'rights talk' and 'cultural talk' in Namaqualand.

Section 1 – Anthropologists and activist strategies: a case of lost in translation?

Activism and indigenous rights

In October 2003 the Constitutional Court had ruled that the Richtersveld community had a legitimate claim to restitution of the land which was being mined by Alexcor, a state-owned diamond mining company. In 2005 the community was back in the Land Claims Court seeking transfer of ownership of the land, loss of income from diamonds mined by Alexcor to the tune of $1.5 billion, environmental damage restitution of R1 billion as well as R10 million in pain and suffering damages (*Mail & Guardian online*, 25 May 2005).[2] In terms of the negotiated settlement outlined in a memorandum in October 2006, the Richtersvelders would withdraw their massive damages claim in return for the transfer of mining rights and the payment of more than R200 million in compensation for the loss of land. The community could then exercise its mining rights by concluding an operation deal with a partner of their choice that could demonstrate capacity (*Mail & Guardian*, 9 March 2007, p. 8).

Although the Richtersveld community was ultimately successful in this restitution case, primordialist conceptions of timeless indigenous culture were deployed

---

[1] Gayatri Spivak's concept of 'strategic essentialism' is used here to refer to the ways in which activists have self-consciously deployed reified and essentialist ideas about indigenous culture and identity in the course of Nama and San land and cultural struggles in the Northern Cape Province (see Chapters 2 and 3 of this book; see also Robins 2001).

[2] *Creamer's Media's Mining Weekly Online* published 25 May 2005 in *Mail & Guardian Online*.

by the state's legal team in an unsuccessful bid to disqualify certain claimants (the *Bosluis Basters*) from benefiting from the claim.[3] The state's legal team argued that the Richtervelders' complicated history of settlement in the Richtersveld prevented a section of the claimant community, the *Bosluis Basters*, from making claims based on indigenous Nama identity. The state's legal strategies were reminiscent of the famous Mashpee Native American Indian case, where the community's expert anthropologist provided a nuanced, historically sensitive account of the complexity of the social construction of 'Mashpee' identity that unwittingly ended up undermining the Native Americans' case (Clifford 1988).

These cases reveal the potential pitfalls of land claims litigation based on indigenous identity. The South African Land Restitution Act does not, however, require that claimants frame their claims in terms of indigenous land rights and cultural identity; they simply have to provide evidence that they were forcibly removed from their land due to racial legislation during the period from 1913 to 1990. Yet, the issue of indigeneity became central to the Richtersvelders' legal arguments, which sought to prove that indigenous Nama-speakers had lived in the area continuously for generations. By framing the land claim in terms of continuous Nama occupation and indigenous identity it was, however, possible for the state's advocate to raise the question as to who was *really* Nama and who was not, and who was feigning Nama membership for material gain. For example, the state's advocate argued that the more recent immigrants into the area, the *Bosluis Basters*, did not qualify because they were *inkomers*, an Afrikaans word used by Namaqualanders to describe those settlers and 'strangers' who come from outside the Coloured Reserves. Advocate Havenga quoted an interview from the doctoral thesis of the Richtersvelders' expert anthropologist, Suzanne Berzborn, in which a 65-year-old Nama man at Kuboes asserted that the claim should only benefit the Nama because it had been their land. The old man said the Basters were claiming that they were Nama through descent on the maternal side in order to access land: 'Now suddenly everyone wants to be Nama, but that is only because of the land claims' (*Mail & Guardian Online*, 4 May 2005).[4] By drawing on Nama identity to buttress the land claim, the Richtersvelders' NGO lawyers from the Legal Resources Centre (LRC) unwittingly created the opportunity for the state's legal team to exploit intra-

---

[3]   When it came to assessing who qualified for hardship and suffering damages, Alexcor's state lawyer questioned the evidence on Nama history and identity led by Cologne University anthropologist, Susanne Berzborn. Advocate Henk Havenga interrogated Berzborn's repeated use, in her doctoral dissertation, of the concept of the 'construction' of Nama identity. Havenga suggested that the community's lawyers had included amongst the claimants the 'Bosluis Basters', an 'assimilated' group of 'Coloured' people of mixed ancestry who, according to the lawyer, had 'invented' themselves as 'Nama' simply because they wanted to access compensation. Berzborn replied that the word construct 'does not not mean invention … What I said in 2000 [in an earlier round of the hearing] and again in my dissertation is that identity is dependent on context' (*Mail & Guardian Online*, 4 May 2005). Following a lengthy process of questioning by Havenga, Geoff Budlender, a member of the Richtersvelders' legal team, told the court that his clients would admit that not everyone and every member of the community suffered in the same way (ibid.).

[4]   Berzborn's response was that the the old man quoted by Havenga was simply the view of one person, and that he was in any case not referring to the Bosluis Basters but rather to other people (*inkomers*) who had come into the Richtersveld from outside the Reserves. Berzborn also argued that the fact that the Bosluis Basters did not speak Nama or want to become Nama was irrelevant as they had a completely different historical background. *Cramer's Media's Mining Weekly Online* published 25 May 2005 in the *Mail & Guardian Online*.

community tensions over questions of Nama identity and cultural authenticity. It also allowed some Nama claimants to use these arguments of ethnic belonging and 'purity' to exclude those considered to be outsiders.

What the Richtersveld case suggests is that resorting to the courts and notions of indigenous rights can result in internal divisions that undermine the cohesion of marginalised communities. A similar situation emerged following the successful ≠khomani San land claim (Chapter 3). For these reasons, there were vigorous debates during the 1970s and 1980s by anti-apartheid activists concerning the strategic efficacy of resorting to rights-based struggles and the courts. It was sometimes argued that litigation contributed towards individualising and fragmenting collective struggles. LRC lawyers were nonetheless able to develop sophisticated modes of legal activism that did not compromise collective struggles against apartheid. During the apartheid years, however, NGOs such as the LRC did not get involved in cultural rights issues but instead focused on racial discrimination and economic concerns.

Whereas indigenous and cultural rights were not prioritised by NGOs and activists during the anti-apartheid struggle, which was framed as a non-racial struggle for national liberation, the post-apartheid period witnessed the growing importance of such rights throughout the world. In South Africa too, the 1990s witnessed indigenous San and Nama groups being increasingly exposed to global indigenous rights discourses. In the 1990s, human rights lawyers such as Henk Smith from the LRC and Roger Chennels from SASI recognised that by stressing indigenous rights and identity, Nama and San communities would gain national and international visibility and support in their land struggles. This visibility was critically important in a post-apartheid context in which hundreds of other communities had submitted land claims to the state for restitution resulting from racially based legislation.

The successful ≠khomani San land claim in the Kalahari District in the Northern Cape Province discussed in Chapter 3 was a direct outcome of the involvement of the South African San Institute (SASI), an NGO that worked on the claim together with the San community. SASI used the media extremely effectively to highlight the claimants' indigenous 'bushman' identity in the build-up to the 1999 land claim. Yet, the San did not win the case on the basis of indigenous land rights, but rather because they were forcibly removed from land in the 1960s as a result of racial legislation. Foregrounding San indigenous identity had nonetheless given the land claim considerable media visibility and political capital. Although in the San case the question of indigeneity was irrelevant from a strictly legal point of view, it helped immeasurably in terms of ensuring that the land claim 'jumped the queue' and was processed in record time.[5] After the community settled on the land, however, serious intra-community divisions emerged between those considered to be authentically San ('the traditionalists') and those labelled as 'outsiders' ('the western bushmen'). Like the Richtersveld case, rights to restitution ended up fuelling contestation over ethnic belonging and cultural authenticity.

Both the ≠khomani San and Richtersveld cases contributed significantly towards

---

[5]   In the Richtersveld case, however, the LRC lawyers introduced indigenous land rights in ways that complicated the legal arguments in the court case itself.

the emergence in the mid-1990s of a vibrant Southern African indigenous rights movement. These successful court cases provided the claimant communities with access to significant land and state resources which they were then able to use to build an indigenous peoples movement. In other words, litigation provided the material means to revitalise and reconstruct forms of indigenous sociality as well as formal institutions and cultural practices. Yet, ironically, the legal issues at stake in the ≠khomani San case had little to do with indigenous rights. The following section discusses these events from the perspective of anthropologists concerned with the ethical and political questions raised by indigenous rights activism in South Africa and elsewhere in the world.

Anthropological conundrums and 'strategic essentialism'

During a field visit to Namaqualand's Leliefontein reserve in the Northern Cape Province in 1996, the earliest accounts of the past I was able to elicit from residents referred to Reverend Barnabas Shaw, the first missionary to arrive at South Africa's first Methodist mission established in 1816. It seemed as if there was a virtual silence about local history prior to Shaw's arrival. The pre-colonial Nama past seemed to have completely vanished from the popular historical imagination. South African anthropologists had explained these silences, and the submergence of Nama identity, by observing that in the past missionised Nama responded to the racist and derogatory connotations that Europeans assigned to the category 'Hottentot' ('Khoi') by distancing themselves from their Nama language and cultural identity and by adopting Afrikaans, Christianity, and the identity of 'Baster' or 'Coloured' (Boonzaier and Sharp 1994).

During the 1980s in Namaqualand, anti-apartheid activists and NGO workers affiliated to the United Democratic Front (UDF) – then regarded as the internal wing of the African National Congress (ANC) – began to realise that indigenous Nama identity could become an important political resource and vehicle for mass mobilisation. These activists set about providing the Nama, 'a people without history' (Wolf 1982), with a politically 'useful past' that connected them to the South African national liberation struggle. As will be discussed below, this also involved grappling with the contradictions between the UDF/ANC activist commitments to rights such as freedom of movement and communitarian notions of Nama belonging (*burgerskap*) and ethnic exclusivity. This activist dilemma could be summed up as the troubling tension between rights and culture. It also raised questions that resonated with Spivak's interrogation of the concept of 'strategic essentialism'.

The South African-born anthropologist, Adam Kuper (2003), has criticised what he regards as the essentialist and undemocratic discourses promoted by NGOs and indigenous rights activists. Kuper argues that these activists are often misguided romantics and partisans who obscure the political dangers of ethnic mobilisation, and fail to address the disjuncture between indigenous identity narratives and the everyday lived realities of those who participate in land claims and indigenous rights movements. For Kuper, 'the realities on the ground' demonstrate that the people these activists work with are usually not nearly as 'authentically indigenous' as activists seem to imply. This position resonates in many respects with Advocate Havenga's argument about the lack of cultural authenticity of the *Bosluis Basters*, who he claimed were simply claiming indigenous identity to benefit from the Richtersveld land claim. Kuper is also concerned that the type of communitarian politics promoted by indigenous rights activists and NGOs tends to create undemocratic politics. NGOs such as *Cultural Survival* come under particular attack for propagating primordialist mythologies of indigeneity that could have 'dangerous political consequences' (2003: 19). According to Kuper, 'since the relative wealth of the NGOs and the locals is so disparate, these movements are unlikely to be democratic' (ibid: 19). In addition, these 'NGO myths' of indigenous identity are used to justify land claims that 'rely on obsolete anthropological notions and on a romantic and false ethnographic vision' (ibid.). Indigenous rights advocates are also blamed for promoting ideologies of 'blood and soil' that share a family resemblance to dangerous and racist European discourses that are routinely used to deny individual rights and justify anti-immigration policies (ibid.). However, surely the essentialising strategies of NGO activists and hyper-marginalised ≠khomani San people in the Kalahari Desert do not compare with forms of xenophobia, chauvinistic nationalism, racism and ethnic cleansing instigated by powerful political parties, nation-states and military forces (see Robins 2003).

Kuper's (2003) criticisms of indigenous peoples' movements are, of course, similar in certain respects to anti-essentialist critiques that are the staple of cultural studies and contemporary anthropology. But the major difference is that Kuper's anti-essentialist critique does not take questions of power and inequality sufficiently seriously. It requires a tremendous stretch of the imagination to compare the 'strategic essentialism' of NGOs and social movements involved in the ≠khomani San land claim with the apartheid state's social engineering policies that resulted in massive social suffering, displacement and political repression in South Africa's ethnic homelands. Whereas activists and NGOs regularly resort to 'benign' forms of strategic essentialism when they represent their clients – female subsistence farmers, female-headed households, the poor, the illiterate, indigenous people, and so on – these forms of essentialism are of a radically different order to the state violence of apartheid social engineering and ethnic cleansing in the Balkans, Rwanda or elsewhere.

Contrary to Kuper's claims, the two chapters in this book on indigenous land and cultural struggles suggest that these constructions of identity by NGOs, activists and indigenous peoples are not in themselves inherently undemocratic or 'politically dangerous'. Neither are they necessarily incompatible with 'rights'. Instead these forms of identity politics often demonstrate a self-conscious reflexivity and ironic engagement with the complexities, ambiguities, cultural hybridities and contradictions that characterise the everyday experiences of marginalised indigenous peoples. Indigenous peoples are regularly required by courts, donors, governments, tourists and anthropologists to conform to these hegemonic logics of cultural authenticity; this may explain why they and their NGO and activist allies are obliged to play the 'essentialising game'. Yet, deploying these forms of strategic essentialism in the courts does not to oblige them to perform their cultural authenticity off-stage, in their everyday lives.

This chapter, as the others that follow, draws attention to the complex ways in which NGO and social movement activists grapple with the competing and situational logics of 'rights talk' and communitarian conceptions of belonging and indigeneity. It also focuses on the ways in which indigenous communities draw on 'things modern' – for instance, state welfare payments, casino royalties and so on – to reconstitute themselves as indigenous peoples. As Marshall Sahlins (1999: ix) notes, the survival of indigenous peoples is often dependent on modern means of production, transportation and communication that they pay for with money acquired from public transfer payments, resource royalties, wage labour, or commercial fishing. Rather than being swallowed up by the homogenising forces of modernity and globalisation, however, many of them recast their dependencies on modern resources and means of production in order to reconstitute their own cultural ideas and practices (1999: ix). Similarly, indigenous groups all over the world are drawing on the resources of a global civil society to reconstitute themselves as 'traditional communities'. Although such processes of cultural reinvention and reconstitution are usually characterised by contradictions and inconsistencies, donors and states often expect these communities seamlessly to perform coherent identities as both Late Stone Age survivors and modern citizens of the nation-state (see Chapter 3).

More anthropological conundrums: critical reflections on 'staged ethnicity'

During the 1980s, anti-apartheid activists focused on populist class-based forms of political mobilisation and popular land struggles rather than on cultural struggles. Intellectuals on the popular left also tended to be dismissive of such cultural struggles (see Boonzaier and Sharp 1993; Mafeje 1971; Magubane 1973). From this neo-Marxist perspective, ethnicity and tribalism constituted forms of 'false consciousness' promoted by the architects of Pretoria's homelands and Separate Development (Bantustan) policies. With the end of apartheid, 'ethnicity' and 'race' replaced 'class' as the keywords of the new official political discourse, and NGOs and indigenous peoples' organisations began to promote self-determination and cultural rights for indigenous peoples. It was in this changing political and intellectual universe that indigenous Nama, San, and Griqua ethnic revitalisation movements took place (see Chapter 3).

In the late 1980s and early 1990s, when discourses on indigeneity first began to surface in the Northern Cape Province, Emile Boonzaier and John Sharp (1994) turned to a constructivist approach to make sense of this dramatic reinvention of Nama identity. Nama 'ethnic revitalisation' was analysed by Boonzaier and Sharp (1994) as 'staged ethnicity' in which carefully controlled and rationally considered performances of Nama identity were part of a repertoire of tactics deployed during the course of land struggles in Namaqualand. In other words, these claims to a Nama past buttressed their legal claims to land in the Reserves. Boonzaier and Sharp supported this argument with their observation that historical legacies of racial discrimination, Christian missionisation and European domination, explained why, until quite recently, Nama history and identity had been so thoroughly submerged. This argument seemed to be confirmed by the apparent disappearance of public expressions of Nama identity following the court case victory.

Boonzaier and Sharp's (1994) analysis implied that behind the Nama mask lies the true face of the assimilated, Westernised and missionised Coloured. However, this perspective failed to acknowledge that cultural hybridity, fragmentation and inconsistency constituted the subaltern condition. The hybrid culture of today's Coloured descendants of the Nama is testimony to the devastation of colonial conquest and domination. This historical experience rendered them incapable of producing the coherent and totalising narratives that are believed to characterise Western histories. In other words, whereas 'the West' is seen to have consistent and convincing history, all the subaltern can aspire to are fragmented fables, origin myths, invented traditions and staged ethnicities. It is precisely because of their shattering encounters with Western domination and ethnocide that the cultural worlds of Namaqualanders consist of fragments, re-inventions, incoherence, disjunctures, silences and hybridity (see Erlmann 1992; Serematakis 1991). This condition reflects and contains the traces and embodied evidence of Nama historical experience.[6] It was precisely by drawing on this shattering historical experience of colonial conquest that the UDF and ANC activists, discussed later in this chapter, were able to reinvent notions of indigenous identity alongside the nationalist discourses of the liberation struggle.

Boonzaier and Sharp's analysis also failed to acknowledge that while the public staging of Nama identity may emerge and recede depending on the political exigencies of the day, Nama memory is also located beyond the domain of public, political life. Fragments of Nama memory inhabit the marginal spaces of everyday social practices, not only the centre-stage of public political arenas. Indeed, it is in these 'off-stage' acts of memory, in the silent shadows of everyday life, that we are likely to find the more deeply inscribed traces of the Nama past. For instance, the traditional structures or *matjieshuise* (mat huts) at the stock posts *(veeposte)*, the fragments of Nama language that are still spoken, the family genealogies and oral narratives, all retain traces of these plundered subaltern identities. These fragments and traces of memory are sometimes recovered and enter the public sphere, as was the case following the court victory and again in the ANC campaigns in the run-up to the April 1994 national elections.

If ambivalence, fragmentation and hybridity are testimony to subaltern experiences of domination, then surely the recovery of these fractured identities is more than simply an instrumentalist act, more than a shrewd and calculated performance of an aboriginal past while living a Westernised and modern present; it is both instrumental and culturally 'authentic' in its reflection of ongoing processes of making meaning of the past. Indeed, it is not a forgery but an act of recuperation and memory. The hybrid appearance of contemporary Nama identity narratives with their amalgam of 'modern' and 'traditional' features reflects the condition of cultural fragmentation that is experienced by subaltern groups elsewhere (see

---

[6] This fragmentation also reflects more recent processes of missionisation, labour migration, urbanisation, and exposure to Western media and educational institutions. However, it is necessary to bear in mind that, despite having had relatively similar experiences, Richtersveld communities in northern Namaqualand have retained considerably more of the Nama language, historical memory and identity than the Afrikaans-speaking Christian residents of Leliefontein. This is probably due to the greater distance of the Richtersveld Reserves from the traditional centres of missionary influence and state control.

Serematakis 1991: 2). The public performances of reclaiming Nama identity were part of a repertoire of cultural and symbolic acts attempting to revive and recover memory. That they were stage-managed and reflected the exigencies of contemporary land struggles in no way rendered them culturally less authentic. Activists and NGO workers involved in these land struggles, as well as those involved in the ≠khomani San land claim discussed in Chapter 3, understood this very well. They also recognised that performing traditional Nama identity did not preclude participating in rights-based struggles over land and citizenship.

The Nama and San case studies suggest that it is extremely unlikely that the 'benign essentialism' and 'staged ethnicity' promoted by indigenous rights NGOs and activists constitute a fundamental threat to democracy, as Kuper would have us believe. It is therefore highly inappropriate to compare ≠khomani San and Inuit identity politics to the violent outbursts of ethno-nationalism, racism, and xenophobia in parts of Europe and Africa. Nonetheless, advocating indigenous Nama identity created real dilemmas for Namaqualand-based NGOs and activists committed to liberal democratic principles. Section 2 of the chapter explores these democratic dilemmas in relation to the attempts by NGOs and activists to reinvent and revive Nama cultural identity in Namaqualand's former Coloured reserves. It investigates the ambiguities and contradictions of the indigenous identity politics promoted by these NGOs and activists. It also argues that this mobilisation of Nama ethnicity in Namaqualand challenges claims that it is purely rational, instrumental or cynical, or that it is simply the recuperation of cultural memory for its own sake. Instead, it would seem that such processes cannot be reduced to singular logics, motivations and intentions. Instead, they reflect the ongoing, and historically situated, reworking of individual and collective political and cultural processes.

Section 2 – NGOs and activists in Namaqualand's Coloured Reserves

Bounded by the Atlantic Ocean to the west and by the Gariep River to the north and bordering on Namibia, Namaqualand falls within the Northern Cape Province, a province with an underdeveloped economic base and the lowest gross domestic product of all the provinces in South Africa. Its economy is dominated by mining and agriculture. The province suffers high levels of poverty, unemployment, crime and violence and infant mortality.

The Namaqualand region is home to six 'Coloured' communal areas – reserves that were designated for people classified as Coloured by the apartheid government.[7] Namaqualand is a sparsely populated, semi-arid region of 47,700 square kilometres and comprises 14 small urban settlements, six Coloured rural areas (the Reserves) and vast tracts of white-owned and mining company land. Almost 50 per cent of the population is employed on the diamond and copper mines, while 9

---

[7]   The six coloured reserves of Namaqualand comprise some 1.7 million hectares of land or 27 per cent of the Namaqualand region, and accommodate about 40 per cent of the region's population (Rohde *et al.* 2001, cited in Lebert 2004: 2). Leliefontein, the southernmost Namaqualand reserve comprises about 190,000 ha (ibid.).

per cent are farm labourers on white farms (Steyn 1989: 416). However, fluctuations in recent years in the copper mining industry have meant that workers are periodically retrenched in large numbers, and the situation has been exacerbated by the closure of smaller mines. In addition, a significant section of the population is employed in the service and manufacturing sectors of the Western Cape as migrant labourers. Many Namaqualand residents, including absent migrant labourers, derive income from the land, primarily as livestock farmers. While wheat, barley, rye and oats are grown, the backbone of the agricultural economy is small stock, goats and sheep, for example. The communal land tenure system in Namaqualand's Reserves has meant that residents have guaranteed access to grazing and arable land. This has provided security for migrant workers who continue to depend on the Reserve, both as a place to retire to and as a safety net in the event of retrenchment.

Many of the inhabitants of Namaqualand are descended from Khoikhoi peoples who have lived in the region for over a thousand years. The history of land dispossession in Namaqualand can be traced to the two Khoikhoi/Dutch wars in 1658-1660 and 1637-1677, and a smallpox epidemic in 1713 that devastated the population (see Boonzaier 1987; Sharp 1977; Steyn 1989). In 1816, Rev. Barnabas Shaw of the Methodist Missionary Society established a mission station in Leliefontein at a time when *trekboers* (migratory farmers of Dutch settler origin) were encroaching onto Namaqua territory. It provided the indigenous population with some degree of protection from the *trekboers*. In 1909 the Mission Station and Reserves Act established the Reserves as communal areas in which tax-paying indigenous Nama people were entitled to graze their animals and cultivate their fields.

The carving up of the communal areas through the development of individual plots or 'economic units' in the 1980s, initiated intense conflict between a relatively small group of 'modernisers' who supported individual tenure, and a considerably larger group of communal farmers who demanded the retention of the communal tenure regime. While the modernisers claimed that individual tenure was a solution to perceived overgrazing and environmental degradation in the Reserves, Leliefontein farmers, together with their NGO and civic activist allies, responded by taking the matter to the Supreme Court in 1988. As a result, communal tenure was reinstated throughout Namaqualand's Reserves.

The economic units proposal had been the outcome of government attempts to promote the growth of a class of better off, educated, small-scale, commercial farmers. Unschooled communal farmers, by contrast, were represented by the apartheid government as environmentally destructive, unproductive and an obstacle to modernisation. Whereas the more schooled and wealthier advocates of individual tenure relied upon discourses of modernisation, individual competition and self-reliance, their opponents (for example, communal farmers, activists, NGOs and human rights lawyers) drew on indigenous (Nama) land claims and discourses on legality, citizenship, rights, democracy and the national liberation struggle. By focusing on fears of land dispossession they addressed the needs of the less educated majority of communal farmers rather than the schooled elite who traditionally dominated local politics.

Proponents of private property, individual tenure and 'progress'
In my interviews with Leliefontein residents in 1994 in the run-up to South Africa's first democratic elections, it became clear that those who reclaimed this indigenous Nama history and identity were perceived to be backward-looking traditionalists by the more educated and better-off local residents who embraced a 'modern' identity as Afrikaans-speaking Christian Coloureds. Proponents of individual tenure and modernisation in the Reserves argued that communal farming was outmoded, unproductive and environmentally destructive. Communal farming, they claimed, was an obstacle to 'progress' and 'development.' They also claimed that Namaqualanders were for the most part thoroughly assimilated and that their claims to a Nama cultural identity were therefore inauthentic, inconsistent and opportunistic (see below). This construction of a 'Great Divide' between tradition and modernity was reproduced 'from above' by the apartheid state as well as 'from below' by better-off farmers seeking access to grazing land through the privatisation of the commons. Chapter 3 discusses a similar divide between 'traditionalists' and 'western bushmen' that surfaced during the post-settlement phase of the ≠khomani San land claim.

Advocates of the need for the modernisation of Namaqualand agriculture included 'Hannes Smit',[8] a retired school principal. For him both Nama culture and communal tenure were obstacles to progress and modernity. Smit substantiated his argument by referring to the influential Theron Commission, an apartheid government report that detailed socio-economic conditions in Namaqualand's Reserves, as well as anthropologist Oscar Lewis's influential 'culture of poverty' thesis. These development ideas were woven into the fabric of locally-embedded religious discourses on individuality and Christian self-reliance, dignity and self-development. Smit represented individual tenure as the antithesis of communal property regimes where dependency on charity and protection from competition were cultivated and reproduced.

> The argument (in the early 1980s) was that people should get rid of the communal system, because it was of no advantage. But people also realised that the communal system is traditional and it is part of the culture of our people. It is therefore not something which can simply be eliminated ... There is something else that really obstructs the development of our community, and it is the culture of poverty which has, over the years, become part of the tradition and lifestyle of our people. If we think that this situation has been given to us by God and you do not see a better situation for yourself, then you just accept it. We hope that through improved education people will escape the spiral of poverty and dependence ... A human being therefore should be responsible for his own progress and this will give him integrity and self-respect. The human being should not have to achieve progress through charity, but by himself with assistance from others. (Interview with H. Smit, March 1994)

Meanwhile, Hannes Smit dismissed Nama identity as not being particularly important in the daily lives of ordinary Leliefontein residents. Echoing the Boonzaier and Sharp's (1994) conception of 'staged ethnicity', he argued that most Leliefontein people were 'modern', and 'Western', and that the emphasis on Nama identity

---

[8] Most of the proper names of interviewees referred to in this chapter are pseudonyms. The names of a few of the better known figures in Leliefontein have not been changed.

in the late 1980s had merely been a short-term tactical manoeuvre to buttress claims to land during the 1988 court case, after which Nama identity vanished from public discourse:

> HS: – The fact that they are Namas has not been emphasised of late. It is not one of the important things anymore. I have listened to people in our meetings and you don't hear it anymore. It has been emphasised a lot when they were still fighting the economic units. They were also proud when the lawyer said to them 'Namas, now you have your land back'. The use of the word Nama is not necessary anymore. They are not proud anymore that they are Nama. They are aware of fashion these days and now the mini [skirt] is out, it has really disappeared. You will for instance still get someone like Japie Bekeur who is one of the big fighters for the rights of the Nama, but he is already an old man. The youngsters do not emphasise that factor about being Nama.
>
> SR: – Are they embarrassed about their Nama ancestry?
>
> HS: – It seems as if this has been a natural death. There are a lot of things which just disappear from life without anybody being aware of it. It seems as if the Nama story does not fit into the present situation anymore.
> (Interview with H. Smit, March 1994)

According to Smit, the younger generations were modernising and striving to secure freehold plots in the cities. This modern orientation, he argued, would eventually trickle down to their 'traditionalist' parents in rural Namaqualand. This representation of a linear and teleological progression led Smit to conclude that Western-style capitalism and individual ownership of land would prevail in the end.

> A modern, Western person believes he needs a title deed for a piece of land. Our children are also struggling in the cities to get a piece of land, while we here are saying no to an opportunity to buy the land ... In Cape Town, if your neighbour has more money than you, he can buy your plot from you. This is a principle of your democratic capitalism of your Western lifestyle. If we want to have the democracy of the Western-world we will have to take the other things as well. (Interview with H. Smit, March 1994)

These narratives of Nama backwardness conform to the taken-for-granted belief that indigenous, minority, or Third World people who display a desire to retain or reclaim aspects of their cultural past constitute an obstacle to development, modernisation and progress.[9] This was endorsed by local Namaqualand elites, who viewed the reclaiming of Nama identity in the 1990s, as well as opposition to the privatisation of the commons, as expressions of peasant conservatism and backward traditionalism.[10] However, whereas Smit made a sharp contrast between tradition and modernity, and anticipated the inexorable march of capitalism as the

---

[9] It has also been widely noted throughout Africa that policy-makers and practitioners regularly refer to concepts such as Hardin's 'tragedy of the commons' thesis, or to Melville Herskovits' characterisation of communal pastoralists in terms of the East African 'cattle complex', to support their claims that adherence to traditions such as communal tenure, or the 'irrational' attachment to cattle, inevitably results in economically unproductive and ecologically destructive agriculture. These development narratives acquire their meaning and salience by drawing on the rhetoric of a 'Great Divide' between modernity and tradition that results in the denial or elision of the hybrid character of many contemporary African identities.

[10] A decade later, however, similar arguments about Nama backwardness were being used to justify the monopolisation of newly acquired commonage by larger and better-resourced reserve farmers to the exclusion of others (Lebert 2004; Wisborg and Rohde 2004). While post-apartheid land redistribution programmes were meant to benefit all communal farmers in Namaqualand, because better-off farmers dominated

final act of this process of development, local responses to economic units were in fact far more diverse.

Activist conceptions of rights and culture in Namaqualand's Reserves

Anti-apartheid and NGO activists mobilised ideas about indigenous Nama identity to challenge state-driven attempts to privatise the commons in Namaqualand's Reserves. These activist interventions challenged 'Great Divide' thinking by splicing local understandings of indigenous Nama identity and historical experience onto a modern African nationalist canvas. This connected Nama identity politics to both popular land struggles elsewhere in South Africa as well as to the national liberation struggle for democratic rights. In their mobilisation of Nama cultural identity in the course of land struggles in Namaqualand, civic activists and NGOs also anticipated the emergence of global indigenous movements that were to take hold in the Northern Cape Province in the latter half of the 1990s amongst people claiming Khoi and San ancestry.

Ideas about Nama cultural identity were mobilised by activists within the context of modern Christian Coloured communities whose memories of their Nama past were in many cases submerged and silent. In addition, the Leliefontein civic activists and NGO development workers who brokered and 're-invented' these ideas about Nama tradition were themselves implicated and enmeshed within liberal modernist discourses and development narratives about linear progress. They were located within structurally ambiguous positions as cultural brokers who mediated 'local' conceptions of indigenous Nama identity and global discourses of development, democracy and progress. This rendered them susceptible to the development ideas advocated by their opponents. For example, while the activists drew on Nama tradition in the 1980s to fight for the reinstatement of communal tenure, they were also sympathetic to development narratives about the alleged ecological destructiveness and unproductive nature of communal livestock systems (see Robins 1994).

In an interview in 1992, 'Manie Cloete', a 38-year-old trade unionist and UDF activist who had been involved in the anti-economic units struggles in the 1980s, stated that he was proud of his Nama ancestry. Yet, Cloete believed that now that communal tenure had been reinstated, traditional farmers had to be educated in order to become modern and market-orientated.

> I think that if people are market-orientated people can get more money [from livestock]. People should also get education on how to be a farmer because our people still depend on traditional ways and means, which I think was actually a good method of doing these things in the past. But now things have changed. I mean, we don't get the amount of rainfall anymore that we used to get in the area. And also there are more and more subsistence farmers, which means that there's this thing of overgrazing ... People don't care about the quality of their stock so that even if you say you're going to be market-orientated you also need to be quality orientated, you see. (Interview with M. Cloete, February 1994)

[10 ctnd] the Commonage Committees they were able to take advantage of the quasi-commercial land use system on the newly acquired muncipal commonage in reserves such as Leliefontein (Lebert 2004: v). Many of those who perceived themselves to be excluded from the benefits of privatisation promoted by elites, defended the character of the commons by once again drawing on arguments about Nama cultural identity.

Given their own position as agents of development and liberal modernism at the margins of the new state, civic activists such as Manie Cloete increasingly found themselves advocating development ideas and practices, such as destocking and fenced paddocks, as well as liberal democratic conceptions of individual rights and freedom of movement, that contradicted and conflicted with those of their rural constituencies.[11] They were drawn to the modernising agendas of those who wished to privatise the commons in order to commercialise agriculture. The changing circumstances of post-apartheid South Africa gave credence and legitimacy to these liberal modernist agendas. These dilemmas were heightened by the recruitment of many former anti-apartheid and NGO activists into the state bureaucracy and development institutions. This created considerable ambiguity amongst activists concerning the value of indigenous knowledge and traditional practices which seemed to contradict the development orthodoxies and democratic credos of modernising ANC elites who were waiting on the sidelines of the new state.

The following section examines how identity narratives mediated access to land in Namaqualand in the 1980s and 1990s. It investigates how these narratives incorporated and reflected upon the social categories of class, occupation, language, and religion, and related these to ideas about Coloured, Nama and Black identities. It will also examine the parameters and limits within which social identities were constructed and contested during the course of land struggles and political mobilisation by activists. While Nama identity narratives and the non-racial nationalist discourses of the ANC mediated by the activists appeared to take hold during the height of the land struggles of the late 1980s and 1990s, it is clear that a modern, conservative Christian Coloured identity continued to provide an extremely powerful sense of belonging and aspiration for many Namaqualanders.

Activist reflections on race, class and Nama identity

Coloured identity in Namaqualand has to be understood within the historical context of colonial conquest, missionisation, miscegenation, apartheid and discourses of nation-building following the April 1994 elections. Coloured Namaqualanders have come to inhabit multiple and shifting identities as Nama (Khoi) Coloureds, *Basters* (people of mixed ancestry – European, Khoi-San, Tswana), Blacks and *Bruin Afrikaners* (Brown Afrikaners). In terms of apartheid's racial classification grid, only Coloureds qualified to live in Namaqualand's Reserves. However, with the end of apartheid and the rise to power of an ANC Government committed to non-racialism, the status of these areas as 'Coloured Reserves' has been challenged.

Manie Cloete spoke from multiple subject positions as a Namaqualander, civic activist, trade unionist and member of the ANC. His trade union background led him to view the land struggles of the 1980s as a class struggle between relatively well-off teachers, business people and local government officials on the one side,

---

[11]   Grazing schemes in communal areas that deploy fenced paddocks are notorious for the conflicts over grazing rights that they engender. In addition, the findings of range ecologists suggest that fenced paddocks are often inappropriate in semi-arid environments since they obstruct the flexibility of livestock movement in a context where key browse resources are widely dispersed across the landscape both spatially and temporally. As a result, these interventions often collide with 'traditional' grazing patterns such as seasonal transhumance.

and activists and communal farmers on the other.

> Ja, within these [Namaqualand] communities there is what you could call a class struggle. The people in the communities don't understand the thing as class struggle, but they know that our teachers and business people practice apartheid here. If I have a shop, or I'm earning a good salary and I have a big house and a car, I will tell my kids not to go and play with those [other] kids because they are not rich. We also find that the wealthy people align themselves with the National Party because they believe that when the ANC takes over, their cars and houses will be taken away from them. It is also this sector of the community that pays their taxes to the Board. Some of them are quite influential, because some of them are [school] principals and so on. (Interview with M. Cloete, February 1994)

Pieter Smit, a 33-year-old Namaqualand-born civic activist, also understood the land struggles in class and occupational terms. As a Leliefontein schoolteacher in the 1980s, Pieter Smit associated with well-educated and better-off residents who, in many cases, also happened to be economic-unit owners. His opposition to the economic units influenced him to leave teaching and devote his energy to working full-time as a civic activist and development worker.

> Poverty was part of my life as a citizen of Leliefontein; nobody is rich here. There was an increase in poverty [and] in diseases like TB. So working in the community made me aware of their problems. And I joined them in their struggle [against economic units]. One part of the community accepted me because I was a teacher who had a [respected] job in the community, and people looked up to me. The poorer people often see teachers, not quite as the enemy, but as people to be afraid of, and who do not freely talk to them. The richer guys, those with a little bit more money than the rest, accept you as their ally. It was those people who had economic units. They were my friends [yet] my personal feeling was that the economic units system was not fair. (Interview with P. Smit, March 1994)

While activists such as Pieter Smit had hoped that participation in the land struggles of the 1980s and early 1990s would encourage Namaqualanders to support the objectives of the national liberation struggle, non-racialism and the class-based politics of the trade union movement, this did not seem to be happening. For the vast majority of Namaqualanders, local land struggles were divorced from national and class politics and instead took on a highly parochial character.

> Not everyone here is interested in what is going on nationally. But if what is decided on the national or even regional level is against their interests, they will stand up as one man and fight that issue. They aren't interested in the national struggle for liberation. They always ask, 'What's going on with these Black people? Why do they kill each other? Why don't they live in peace?' But the Namaqualanders have had their own struggles. (Interview with P. Smit. March 1994)

Both Pieter Smit and Manie Cloete were activists committed to the ANC's ideologies of non-racialism and liberal modernism, but this did not prevent them from also being drawn to a Nama past and a Nama cultural identity. Their challenge was to somehow wed these ethnic particularist identities to the ANC's liberal democratic political project. Cloete identified as a Namaqualander and an 'ANC person,' but also took pride in his *Baster* and Khoi ancestry:

> MC: – Basically, a *Baster* is a child of a Nama and a White person. In all these years there's lots of people like me, *Basters*. A Nama person will maybe marry a *Baster* and so on. But if

you're not having these Khoi features, you're not a Nama. It's very interesting to sit down with people and actually ask them, 'How do you know that I am a *Baster* or a Khoi?' Then also your hair and colour of your eyes and these things will also play a role, you see ... For myself, I identify myself as being a Namaqualander. This thing about *Baster* and Khoi is not so important for me. I mean, my mother was a *Baster* and my father originated from Khoi. So I don't have a problem. For me, I can go to Nama people and they will accept me. I can go to *Baster* people and sometimes I get more problems from them. Sometimes there's more acceptance from the so-called Nama people than from the *Baster* people due to the fact that I'm also a prominent ANC person. So I sometimes am more accepted by the Nama people because I identify myself with their problems, with their experiences. While your sort of *Baster* people see themselves as an elite group of people.

SR: – Are you proud of being Nama?

MC: – Ja. The thing that I'd really like to do in future is learn Nama. But the Nama language is only spoken by a few people.

(Interview with M. Cloete, February 1994)

While activists such as Cloete were drawn to a Nama identity, they were wary of Namaqualanders' parochialism, racism and ethnic exclusivism, attitudes which clashed with the ANC's 'non-racial' liberal modernism. Despite an apparent nostalgia for a lost Nama language and culture, activists such as Manie Cloete and Pieter Smit defined themselves first and foremost as South Africans and members of the ANC, a non-racial political organisation with both liberal and socialist ideological orientations. They had anticipated and hoped that political mobilisation around popular land struggles would bring Namaqualand's Nama Coloured residents closer to Black South Africans and the ANC. However, they found that events of the 1980s and 1990s had in fact reinforced parochialism and 'insiderism'. Divisions between insider *burghers* (citizens, that is Coloured Namaqualanders) and *inkomers* (White, Black or Coloured outsiders) remained, and in response to the uncertainty of the 1990s, local Coloured elites were again calling for individual tenure, this time to pre-empt possible plans to open the Reserves to landless Blacks (i.e. Africans). As a result, many Namaqualanders continued to fear that the Reserves would be 'invaded' by Blacks.

Prior to 1990, non-Coloureds had to obtain permits in order to visit the Reserves. Manie Cloete believed that fear and mistrust of *inkomers,* especially Black South Africans, had intensified with the demise of apartheid.

People are even having a problem with White people (coming here). We discussed this with our civic earlier last year, when the Councils wanted the land to be reserved for Coloured people. They actually sent resolutions to the land conference, also to the House of Representatives. They demanded that the so-called Reserves must be kept for so-called Coloured people. And we had this debate. Some of our kids go to Cape Town or Johannesburg, and meet a White man or White girl, or a Black man or a Black girl, and they fall in love, and want to get married. Now what is the position then going to be? Must I then allow my daughter to bring a Black husband to Concordia [Reserve] or whatever the case should be? So these things are taking place in practice. Everyday people are starting to realise that this is not something that we are going to stop ... The civics [must] educate people that if a Black man or a White man wants to come and stay in Concordia, he's welcome. But he must just fall in with the norms within the community. That is basically what we want. We don't want our land to be sold. We

> don't want someone to come in and buy a big piece of land because we want to keep it as communal. So if someone, never mind his colour, wants to come and stay in Concordia, he must just fit in with the norms that we practise in the community. (Interview with M. Cloete, February 1994)

Given the freedom of movement provisions in the post-apartheid Constitution, Namaqualanders are unable to deny Black Africans the right to settle in the former Coloured Reserves. Yet, in the early 1990s the prospect of an influx of Blacks into the area generated considerable debate and trepidation. Proponents of individual tenure responded to this new situation by calling for tenure reform as a means of protecting and securing land owned by Namaqualanders from possible future claims of Black settlers. Cloete challenged rumours of a 'black invasion' yet they kept resurfacing. His own experiences as a UDF activist made him familiar and comfortable with the ideology of non-racialism, and, as a trade union organiser, he envisaged the possibility of Black and Coloured working-class solidarity. Yet, his upbringing in Namaqualand forced him to confront the reality and resilience of Coloured identity and of local discourses on racial difference.

> You see, most of the communities in Namaqualand are Afrikaans-speaking, and also because of apartheid Blacks used to live in compounds. For example, when I was a little kid, when I used to be a bit naughty my mother would tell me, 'Look, *daar kom die kaffir en die kaffir gaan jou vang'* (here comes the kaffir and he's going to catch you). So as from childhood we were actually scared of Africans. [Then] what happened was that in the unions it was not so difficult to get the people to understand what racism was about. Because, I mean, Blacks and Coloureds used to work together. They used to receive the same treatment from the company, although the Black people received much harsher treatment. But there was this relationship between Coloured workers and Black workers, [who] are actually often fluent in Afrikaans. If you go to De Beers mines and you ask Black workers how long they have been working there, they will say up to 20 or 25 years. So there's this relationship ... But some of our people are even more racist than Whites. Actually, it will be a long struggle and long fight to educate people [that] we're all human beings ... Education is going to play an important role. (Interview with M. Cloete, February 1994)

Activist mediations of identity politics during the transition to democracy

During the 1994 elections ANC activists focused on fusing accounts of Nama colonial conquest and land dispossession with a national liberation narrative. 'Chris September', a Coloured, ANC activist, addressed questions of Nama cultural identity, colonialism and apartheid at a meeting in 1994 to launch a Namaqualand ANC branch. In his speech he constructed an elaborate web of cultural and historical connections between the experiences of oppression of Black South Africans and the history of the Nama, Khoikhoi and San. The audience were mostly Namaqualanders many of whom had over the years come to see themselves as Coloureds, *Bruin Mense* or *Bruin Afrikaners*. Despite these experiences of fragmentation and cultural amnesia, September sought to resuscitate historical memory of a Khoikhoi past and provide a coherent anti-colonial narrative that would have salience for both Namaqualanders and the ANC.

> We have suffered a great injustice during the years of apartheid and colonialism. Number one, we lost our language. And language is a powerful weapon because it binds people and makes

them one. We lost our language. In the old Khoikhoi language there were about 20 dialects or regional languages which we spoke with 16 clicks ... The Xhosa people got their clicks from us ... The White people came. They took our language away from us, and with that they took the greatest part of our culture from us. The second thing they took was our land. In the old Khoikhoi tradition no person owned land... The land belonged to all of us. (Speech by C. September, March 1994)

September then went on to provide a history of the Khoikhoi and San people and described how slavery, colonialism and apartheid had destroyed their religion, culture and language. His account of the legacy of colonial conquest attempted to revive collective memory amongst a people who appeared to have lost sight of their Nama identity and Nama past. It sought to reinvent a local Nama identity and splice it onto a national liberation narrative.

People like to say that the Khoikhoi people who lived around here had never known God and his commandments. Maybe we didn't have their beautiful churches and their bibles. But our people knew God. *Tiqua* was the name of our God and is still the name of our God. Now when you are ruined and have lost your religion you become *Na!wu*, which means we were finished, and there was nothing left of us. And then the church came and saved us from being *Na!wu*, and made us people again. The reason why I am sketching this for you, my brothers and sisters, comrades, is so that I can tell you that the struggle against ... injustice isn't a struggle which began yesterday. It is a struggle which began when we lost our culture and our land, when we lost our cattle, when we lost our humanity. And that's what happened when they came to take over our land. (Speech by C. September. February 1994)

The rest of September's speech was concerned with an indictment of racism and exploitation, explaining why the ANC launched the armed struggle, allaying fears that the communist influence in the ANC was a threat to religious freedom, and assuring Namaqualand residents that the Bill of Rights protected the property, cultural, religious and language rights of all citizens: 'So should someone call you a *Hotnot* [Hottentot],[12] you can take him to court'. He also assured everyone present that no outsiders *(inkomers)* had a right to interfere in local agriculture and land matters: 'Nobody will touch our ground. No one touches our herds.' September's speech had spliced together Nama, Coloured and religious themes and identities and incorporated these into a coherent national liberation narrative. This hybrid discursive framing no doubt contributed to the success of ANC and NGO activists in the land struggles of the 1980s, as well as the ANC Northern Cape victories in national and local government elections since 1994.

The reinvention of Nama identity in Leliefontein in the early 1990s seemed to some to have been a short-lived tactical move deployed by UDF and ANC activists and communal farmers for the purpose of litigation and mobilisation for the 1994 national elections. Yet, two decades later, there was still an indigenous rights movement in South Africa. The public performances of Nama identity in the 1980s and 1990s also appear at first glance to be a variation of Hobsbawm and Ranger's (1983) 'invention of tradition' thesis. However, these 'Nama inventions' emerged from dialogic encounters between NGO and activist cultural brokers and communal farmers, rather than being simply imposed 'from above' (see Jeannerat 1995).

---

[12] *Hotnot* is a derogatory Afrikaans term used to refer to Hottentot (Khoikhoi) and Coloured people.

In other words, the Namaqualand case could be seen as an example that highlights the agency and creativity of those for whom traditions are usually seen to be 'invented'.

Aspects of this form of cultural invention could perhaps best be described as a form of strategic essentialism from below. This does not mean, however, that these 'invented traditions' were simply forgeries or faked copies of originals deployed for purely instrumental purposes. Instead, their resurfacing in the 1980s and 1990s land struggles reflected the fragmentation, disjunctures, hybridity and absences of the subaltern condition. The discrepancies, gaps and silences were themselves the products of colonial and apartheid violence and domination. It was indeed these buried transcripts of the past that the ANC activist, Chris September, excavated and brought to the surface in his election campaign speech in Namaqualand in 1994. September's speech wove a discursive thread between these traces of 'local' Nama historical experience and the broader contours of a modernist national liberation struggle.

Prior to the elections, Namaqualanders were represented by journalists and pollsters as Coloured Christian conservatives.[13] In terms of these representations, they not only shared a common language and cultural identity with White Afrikaners, but were equally suspicious and racist towards Black Africans *(Mail & Guardian*, 13 May 1994). While there may have been some substance to aspects of this portrayal, it failed to account for the fact that many Coloured Namaqualanders, especially those in the northern parts of the Richtersveld, voted for the ANC and identified with the national liberation narrative. The ANC's electoral successes in the Northern Cape since 1994 were probably due to the support that NGOs and community-based organisations, aligned with the United Democratic Front (now the ANC) gave to poorer communal farmers in the land struggles discussed in this chapter. The vast tracts of land redistributed to communal farmers by the ANC government during the first decade of democracy no doubt also played a significant role in these electoral successes. These successes were also due to the intimate connections that anti-apartheid activists and NGOs were able to forge between Nama and Black South African historical experiences of land, linguistic and cultural dispossession.

Conclusion

During the land struggles of the 1980s, the mobilisation of Nama identity of necessity took on an inclusive character (see Boonzaier 1996; Sharp 1994). Most residents in the thoroughly missionised Leliefontein Reserve did not speak

---

[13] Prior to the April 1994 national elections, many Coloured Namaqualanders had also expressed strong opposition to rumours that Namaqualand would be incorporated into a right-wing Afrikaner *volkstaat* (homeland) or become part of a Conservative Party-dominated Northern Cape. There were demands for a referendum to test whether Namaqualanders wanted to be part of the Northern or Western Cape. People I interviewed before the elections claimed that they would choose to be part of the Western Cape. By winning 50 per cent of the Northern Cape vote, the ANC took many by surprise and laid to rest fears of the *volkstaat* scenario. The election result also defied predictions that Coloureds in the Northern Cape. who comprised 54 per cent of the region's population, would vote Nationalist Party en bloc.

Nama any longer, and Nama history had been all but forgotten.[14] It was therefore hardly surprising that activists promoted forms of political mobilisation in which the boundaries of Nama belonging were permeable, negotiable and inclusive. However, contrary to postmodern conceptions of social identities as infinitely indeterminate and open-ended, civic activists recognised that social and economic location significantly shaped local attitudes towards both communal tenure and the parameters within which identities were constructed in Leliefontein. Activists also believed, with some justification, that mobilising indigenous identity in Namaqualand would not necessarily prevent Nama communal farmers from also identifying as modern rights-bearing citizens. These mobilisation experiences learnt in Namaqualand revealed the changing nature of political mobilisation in the transition to democracy.

By drawing on Nama identity, these Afrikaans-speaking, Christian Coloureds and their NGO and activist allies were not calling for a return to some pristine and primordial Nama past. Theirs was not simply a traditionalist response by people claiming to be descendants of the Nama. After all, their response included intimate engagement with legal and bureaucratic practices of the modern state, as well as modernist discourses on national liberation, the law (*die wet*), rights, citizenship, development and democracy.

Activists within NGOs and anti-apartheid political organisations[15] played a crucial role in facilitating what Boonzaier and Sharp (1994) refer to as the rediscovery of Nama identity in the 1980s and 1990s. These activist brokers were not motivated by a desire to revive or preserve a timeless and exotic indigenous culture, but were attempting to connect ideas about Nama tradition with liberal modernist struggles for democracy and rights. By linking the fragments of local cultural worlds to the discourses of the national liberation struggle, these *bricoleurs* (Levi-Strauss 1966) and cultural brokers (Geertz 1960; Wolf 1966) managed to mobilise support for the ANC in many parts of Namaqualand. At the same time, they mediated local access to complex legal and bureaucratic literacies, institutional practices, and discourses on citizenship and rights.

This resistance to individual tenure was not simply a local response based on nostalgia for Nama tradition. Neither was this opposition simply the outcome of a parochial, 'ethnic' politics of autochthony (Geschiere and Nyamnjoh 2002). Instead, it emerged out of land struggles that drew on both modern discourses – on rights, citizenship, democracy and national liberation – as well as indigenous histories and identities that had been shattered and silenced through colonial domination and apartheid. Furthermore, the diverse and hybrid tactics and repertoires that were evident during these land struggles were indicative of the more generalised conditions of cultural hybridity, contingency, improvisation and instability of Coloured identity and marginalised people in South Africa and elsewhere. These

---

[14] Some of the older Leliefontein residents knew the original Nama names of certain places in the area, and traditional Nama *matjieshuise* (round huts) continue to be built. Nama is widely spoken in the Richtersveld area near the Namibian border.

[15] These activists and development workers belonged to the United Democratic Front (later the ANC). The National Union of Mineworkers (NUM) and anti-apartheid NGOs such as the Surplus People Project (SPP) and the Legal Resources Centre (LRC).

land and cultural struggles expressed a hybrid political logic that collapsed the artificial binary between rights and culture. Furthermore, these moral and political dilemmas did not constitute a threat to democracy and rights along the lines anticipated by Adam Kuper in his critique of indigenous rights activism. The dramatic rise and decline of the public performance of Nama identity demonstrated the capacity of Leliefontein residents to deploy a 'benign,' heterogeneous and hybrid repertoire of tactics in their engagement with the rapidly shifting terrain of South African national politics. This was a far cry from the ethno-nationalist 'blood and soil' politics of apartheid, the Balkans and Rwanda.

While Nama identity was visible and had salience in Leliefontein in the 1980s, the political mobilisation after the April 1994 elections brought to the fore contestations over Coloured, Black and *Bruin Afrikaner* identity. The public performance of Nama identity seemed to recede after the elections but this did not mean that Nama identity politics had completely disappeared. It continued in the form of a relatively small indigenous rights movement based largely in the Northern Cape Province. It also remained inscribed in the *matjieshuise* (traditional Nama structure usually made from grasses and other veld material) and oral narratives, and its residual cultural elements were readily available for the creative manipulations of activist bricoleurs and NGO brokers who sought to link these local cultural forms to broader national concerns. Nama cultural continuity expressed in vernacular architecture and oral histories provided material for connecting this historical memory to a meta-history of the liberation struggle in South Africa. It also provided the political, cultural and symbolic capital for an indigenous rights movement that was waiting to be inaugurated in the 'new' South Africa. With the persistance of land struggles and tensions between elite and poorer communal farmers in Namaqualand, these competing discourses on modern *Baster*/'Coloured'/*Bruin Afrikaner* and 'traditonal' Nama identity continue to frame contemporary political discourses (see Lebert 2004; Wisborg and Rohde 2003). The following chapter on the cultural politics of land and ≠khomani San identity in the Kalahari follows on from this account of the first rumblings of a post-apartheid indigenous people's movement.

Acknowledgements

The chapter is part of work carried out within the Project on Civil Society, Department of Political Studies, Witwatersrand University and the Albert Einstein Institute. Some of the research for this chapter was also part of work done within the Social Uses of Literacy Project (SOUL), Department of Adult Education at the University of Cape Town. I would also like to thank Ben Cousins, Allen Feldman, Jeff Lever, Pat McAllister, Martin Prinsloo, Tom Lodge and Henk Smith for comments. I would also like to thank Lala Steyn, Fiona Archer and Harry May of the Surplus People Project, Llewellyn Links, Louis van Wyk and many other Leliefontein residents for their generous support and assistance.

Interviews
Ben Bezuidenhout, Leliefontein, March 1994.

Gert Bekeur, Leliefontein, February 1994, September 1994, March 1996.
'Hannes Smit', Karkams, March 1994.
'Manie Cloete', Springbok, February 1994.
Pieter Smit, Leliefontein, March 1994, September 1994, March 1996.

Speech
'Chris September', Leliefontein, March 1994.

3

Citizens & 'Bushmen'
The ≠khomani San, NGOs
& the Making of a New Social Movement

November 21, 2004 will go down in history as the day that *Hoodia gordonii* was 'discovered' in America. It was on that date that CBS 60 Minutes aired a program about *Hoodia gordonii* and for the first time many people were introduced to this traditional botanical product. Now word of this amazing product is spreading like wildfire and taking the consumer market by storm. Many are calling the medical discovery of *Hoodia gordonii* the greatest breakthrough in weight loss management of the decade! *Hoodia gordonii* is the plant with the new wonder ingredient that curbs one's appetite and helps one to slim. *Hoodia gordonii* is a succulent plant from the Kalahari Desert, home of the San people. The San have been using the *Hoodia gordonii* succulent for centuries to stave off hunger during their long and arduous hunting trips in the harsh South African wild. Now you too can lose weight with this miracle diet pill. The discovery of the active ingredient in the *Hoodia gordonii* plant is proven with clinical research to suppress one's appetite by up to 2000 calories a day. This amazing and all natural and organic ingredient is the result of 30 years of research by the CSIR (Council for Scientific and Industrial Research) in South Africa. So great is the discovery of this weight-loss ingredient that Pfizer, a large pharmaceutical company, is developing a pill, known as P57, based on the *Hoodia gordonii* plant. Why does Pfizer need to synthesise a product that already works you may ask? In America you cannot patent a natural product so the drug companies need to turn it into a drug by making an unnatural and unhealthy substance so they can patent the product and make billions of dollars. We are delighted to report that WIMSA contested and recently won their case against multinational pharmaceutical companies seeking to develop a drug from South African *Hoodia*. (Internet search for *Hoodia gordonii: www.google.Hoodia* Gordonii Plus-files, 2007/03/15, 14:17)

Following their successful land claim in 1999, the ≠khomani San's lawyer, Roger Chennels, successfully negotiated an agreement with Pfizer, an international drug giant that was interested in San indigenous knowledge and traditional use of *Hoodia gordonii*, a plant that the company wished to use to manufacture and market internationally as an appetite-suppressant called P57. The San had apparently chewed this cactus plant for generations to suppress their thirst and appetite during long hunting trips in the parched Kalahari Desert. Given the international demand for anti-obesity drugs, the market for P57 could run to billions of dollars.[1]

---

[1]   In terms of the deal, the South African Council for Scientific and Industrial Research (CSIR) will pay

51

This historic agreement followed a regrettable remark by a Pfizer representative that the San had once used *Hoodia* but that they were now extinct. This comment was in response to questions by journalists as to whether the San could expect compensation for their contribution to the 'discovery' of this new drug.[2] By 2006 *Hoodia*-derived slimming products were being marketed throughout the world, in most cases without any recognition of San intellectual property rights.[3]

Petrus Vaalbooi, a ≠khomani San leader in the Kalahari District of the Northern Cape Province, appeared in Rehad Desai's *Bushmen's Secret* documentary as the signatory of a multi-million rand *Hoodia* deal that promised to provide the ≠khomani San with a massive source of revenue generated from the international marketing of *Hoodia*. Although Vaalbooi appeared at the signing ceremony dressed in 'traditional' bushman skins and loincloths, when I first met him in 1999 he only wore western clothing, and was labelled by 'traditionalists' in his community as an assimilated 'western' bushman. At the time there were deep divides between the 'traditional' and 'western' bushmen. Six years later, Vaalbooi was appearing regularly in public looking like a truly 'traditional' bushman. Desai's documentary also told the story of another man, Jan van der Westhuizen, a traditionalist who makes a living as a San traditional healer. In a disturbing scene, Elias Le Riche, the former white warden whose family have run the Kalahari National Park since the early decades of the last century, tells Desai and Van der Westhuizen on camera that he knows for certain that Van der Westhuizen is not a 'real' bushman. He claims to know all of the 'real' bushmen' of the Kalahari. Van der Westhuizen is silent and seems devastated by this judgement. Turning to Dawid Kruiper, a well-known ≠khomani San leader, Le Riche affirms the pedigree of the Kruiper family as 'the real thing'. He seems to have no qualms assuming the position of ultimate arbiter of 'bushman' authenticity.

For Nigel Crawhall, a San linguist who heads up the South African San Institute's (SASI) culture and heritage management programme, the *Hoodia*-drug deal offered the prospect of providing the financial means to salvage what remained of San culture, language and identity, which had been all but destroyed as a result of violent encounters with colonialism, capitalism and apartheid. Prior to the land claim and the *Hoodia* deal, the ≠khomani San had lived scattered throughout the sparsely populated and underdeveloped Northern Cape Province of South Africa working as farm labourers and living off welfare grants in impoverished rural and urban ghettoes. *Hoodia* seemed to offer the possibility of reversing the trajectory of these devastating historical processes of dispossession, dislocation, impoverishment and marginalisation.

Although the land the ≠khomani San won through the restitution process had not generated any significant income, Chennels' deft legal footwork on cultural and intellectual property rights, together with the success of SASI's culture, language

---

1 ctnd the San 8 per cent of payments made by its licensee, UK-based Phytopharm, during the drug's clinical development phase. The biggest revenue stream could come from 6 per cent royalties the San would receive if and when the drug is marketed by Pfizer.
2 Leon Marshall, 'Africa's Bushmen May Get Rich From Diet-Drug Secret'. *National Geographic News*, April 16, 2003.
3 See Rehad Desai's documentary on *Hoodia* entitled *Bushmen's Secret*. Desai shows how the plant is being used by the pharmaceutical industry to manufacture products that do not in any way benefit the San.

and heritage programmes, had created a lucrative San brand. The inspiration for this international San brand name came from Australian Aborigines who had succeeded in marketing tourist packages that involved travelling thousands of kilometres through the Australian desert to see the authentic indigenous sacred sites. This model was now being used to promote cultural tourism to the ≠khomani San settlement which is adjacent to the Kalagadi Transfrontier Park (Chennels, personal communication). This commodification of San culture, heritage and indigenous knowledge, that John and Jean Comaroff call *Ethnicity Inc.* (see Comaroff & Comaroff forthcoming), revealed new ways in which NGO lawyers and activists were using cultural and intellectual property rights to assist marginalised communities to access donor, state and big business dollars. These substantial resources were in turn being used to constitute new forms of indigenous culture, sociality and collective identity. These legal interventions, commercial ventures and rights claims did not automatically translate into the kinds of individualism and depoliticisation anticipated by critics of rights-based NGOs and social movements. Instead, they provided the material infrastructure and possibilities for the resuscitation and 'reinvention' of indigenous cultural forms and practices from the debris, fragments and burial grounds produced by colonial violence and histories of dispossession.

The previous chapter focused on the complex and ambiguous roles of NGOs and anti-apartheid activists involved in the 'reinvention' of Nama identity and the embryonic phase of the making of an indigenous peoples movement in Northern Cape Province in the late 1980s and early 1990s. The chapter shows how these activists and NGOs mediated new indigenous modernities that sought to reconcile notions of indigenous Nama identity and liberal individualist conceptions of the rights-bearing modern citizen. Following the April 1994 democratic elections these developments intensified with the establishment of land restitution programmes that sought to return land to black South Africans who were dispossessed as a result of racial land laws. In addition, the new post-apartheid constitution protected cultural and language rights, and the state earmarked funding for the development of indigenous languages. These developments, together with Thabo Mbeki's vision of an African Renaissance and the United Nation's declaration of the 1990s as the Decade of Indigenous Peoples Rights, were catalysts for NGO and community-based mobilisations around indigenous land, cultural and language rights. Given these developments, it is not surprising that the first decade after apartheid was also a period of litigation and political contestation over liberal individualist conceptions of rights versus collective notions of cultural rights and customary law (see Comaroff and Comaroff 2005). It was within this shifting terrain of political, legal and cultural struggles that the ≠khomani San land claim was lodged with the Land Claims Court.

Land claims, indigenous movements and their critics

During the ≠khomani San land claim process of the mid-1990s, the claimants were regularly represented on television documentaries and in the print media as a highly cohesive and consensual community with a common cultural heritage and continuity. Media representations of the San land claim process comprised a series of stereotypical images of timeless and primordialist San 'tribes' reclaiming their ancestral land. Deputy President Thabo Mbeki's speech on the 22 March 1999 at the Human Rights Day celebration of the signing of the historic land restitution agreement was optimistic that the return of the land to the ≠khomani San would heal the wounds of the past. Mbeki spoke of the dreams of a return from exile for the ≠khomani San claimants who had been scattered across the Northern Cape living in rural ghettoes and in poverty-stricken conditions in communal areas and on white farms:

> We shall mend the broken strings of the distant past so that our dreams can take root. For the stories of the Khoe and the San have told us that this dream is too big for one person to hold. It is a dream that must be dreamed collectively, by all the people. It is by that acting together, by that dreaming together, by mending the broken strings that tore us apart in the past, that we shall produce a better life for you who have been the worst victims of oppression.

Subsequent to the successful resolution of the land claim in 1999, these optimistic bushman images and narratives were replaced by front-page *Cape Times* reports of conflict, homicide, suicide, alcohol abuse, AIDS, and social fragmentation at the new San settlements in the Andriesvale-Askam area adjacent to the Kalahari Gemsbok National Park (KGNP), Northern Cape Province. In early 2004 the South African Human Rights Commission began an inquiry into human rights violations and the abject conditions of the Kalahari San. The commission had received complaints of the murder of a community member by the police, as well as allegations of police victimisation and harassment. There were also complaints about community divisions and 'the involvement of too many external consultants, NGOs and other parties' in ≠khomani San matters. In addition, community members complained about the government's failure to provide services and to support the community in the land resettlement progress.[4] Newspapers also reported on allegations of financial mismanagement by the ≠khomani San Communal Property Association (CPA) and the dire consequences for the community of divisive leadership struggles.[5]

A striking aspect of these conflicts was the emergence of intra-community tensions between the self-designated 'traditionalists' and the 'western' bushmen at the new settlement area. This divide drew on markers of cultural authenticity that included genealogies, language, 'bush knowledges', bodily appearance, clothing and so on. These tensions, only a year after the land signing ceremony, raised a number of troubling questions: How come what was widely perceived to be a cohesive and 'harmonious' San community had so quickly come to be seen as a deeply fractured group of individuals struggling to constitute themselves as a community? Was the notion of San community and solidarity a strategic fiction fashioned by the San and their NGO allies during the land claims process? What happened in the

---

[4] *Report on the Inquiry into Human Rights Violations in the Khomani San Community*, South African Human Rights Commission, November 2004, p. 5.
[5] *Cape Times*, 5 May 2000.

post-settlement phase to unleash processes that undermined this prior appearance of solidarity? How could one explain the dramatic shift from media celebrations of a pristine and consensual hunter-gatherer culture in March 1999, to the more sober, and at times quite grim, journalistic descriptions of the Kalahari San settlement a year later? Finally, why did local constructions of a 'great divide' between traditional and western bushmen emerge when they did?

In attempting to answer these questions I became increasingly interested in the roles of non-governmental organisations (NGOs) in local political processes, in mediating representations of the San, and in brokering global discourses on civil society, cultural survival and indigenous peoples rights. Fieldwork encounters in the Kalahari San settlement in 1999 drew my attention to the effects of these donor and NGO discourses on local constructions of community, cultural authenticity and identity in the Kalahari. It appeared that, despite these local constructions of a 'great divide' between traditionalists and western bushmen, none of the Kalahari San fitted the mould of indigenous people untouched by modernity, neither were they modern citizens completely moulded by discourses of western democracy and liberal individualism. Instead San identities, local knowledges and everyday practices were composed of hybrid discourses. This begged the question as to how this great divide had emerged.

This line of inquiry raised further questions concerning the impact of the contradictory objectives of NGOs and donors to both: provide support for traditional leadership, San language and cultural survival, and inculcate modern/western ideas and practices of democratic decision-making, accountability, and the civic virtues of rights, duties and responsibilities. It began to appear as if the traditionalist versus western bushman dichotomy in the Kalahari was itself partly a result of this contradiction and ambiguity at the heart of donor and NGO development agendas. Could these donor *double visions* of the San – as both 'First Peoples' and citizens-in-the-making – be a catalyst for these intra-community divisions? This chapter investigates how these global discourses on communitarian indigeneity and liberal democracy were brokered by an NGO, the South African San Institute (SASI), and re-appropriated and reconfigured from below by San communities. It draws attention to the ambiguities and contradictions embedded within these development discourses on San tradition and civic citizenship, and examines how this contributed towards intra-community divisions and leadership struggles within a hyper-marginalised ≠khomani San community. These leadership struggles and divisions also draw attention to the problematic ways in which notions of San tradition and First People status can be deployed as strategies of exclusion that promote intra-community division. It appeared that, despite the thoroughly hybridised character of contemporary San identity, knowledges and practices, San traditionalists sought to stabilise bushman identity through recourse to notions of a detribalised Other, the 'western bushmen' living in their midst. These processes of intra-community conflict, which surfaced shortly after the San were settled on their newly acquired land, followed a highly successful land claim process that had highlighted notions of San traditionality.

The hybridised conditions of everyday life in the Kalahari includes 'local' knowledges, practices and identities as well as San access to exogenous cyber-technologies, fax machines, cellular phones and international indigenous peoples' conferences and conventions in Europe and North America. This hybridity draws attention to the existence of what some scholars refer to as indigenous moderni-ties (Gupta 1998; Povinelli 1999 a and b; Sahlins 1999) that challenge traditional versus modern dichotomies. This chapter aims to bring these theoretical debates to a growing literature on San histories and identities in southern Africa,[6] and a less developed one on the relation between indigenous people, NGOs and civil society in Africa (Garland 1999). It also aims to contribute towards studies of the cultural politics of land restitution in South Africa after apartheid (James 2000a and b; Robins 2000).

The cultural politics of indigenous identity discussed in this chapter only became publicly visible in South Africa in the 1990s. Unlike the situation of indig-enous groups such as the Pan-Mayan Movement in Guatemala, where about 60 per cent of the population are said to have an indigenous background, San and Nama 'ethnic revitalisation' has been confined to relatively small numbers of people mostly from the Northern Cape Province. The South African San Institute (SASI) was established in the early 1990s as the first, and only, NGO in South Africa dealing with indigenous issues. SASI was established by a human rights lawyer, Roger Chennels, who, in the late 1980s, became involved in attempts to negotiate improved labour conditions for San farm workers at the Kagga Kamma bushman tourist village at Ceres, a few hundred kilometres from Cape Town (White 1995). Chennels soon realised that the ≠khomani San community was in a strong posi-tion to succeed in a land claim. Since the San had been forcibly removed from the Kalahari Gemsbok National Park (KGNP), as a direct result of racial legislation implemented after the 1913 cut-off date period, their claim would be taken seri-ously by the Commission for Land Rights and Restitution. The preparations for the land claim initiated a process of San cultural 'revitalisation' that was later to be spearheaded by SASI.

During the 1980s, anti-apartheid activists and rural NGOs had focused on populist class-based forms of political mobilisation and popular land struggles rather than cultural struggles. These NGOs were often affiliated with the United Democratic Front (UDF) and formed part of a broad Left coalition of trade unions and civic organisations. Intellectuals in the popular Left tended to be dismissive

---

[6] There is a vast literature on San communities in Namibia and Botswana that addresses similar issues to the South African situation. Examples of this extensive literature include Lee, R., 1979, *The !Kung San*; Wilmsen, E., 1989, *Land Filled with Flies: A Political Economy of the Kalahari*; Gordon, R., 1992, *The Bushman Myth and the Making of a Namibian Underclass*. This chapter, however, will be restricted to the case of a specific San community in the Northern Cape Province in South Africa. The following references draw attention to a burgeoning literature on Khoi and San issues in South Africa: Boonzaier, E., 1992, 'Rediscovering the Nama: a Case Study of Controlled Identity Politics in the North-West Cape', chapter presented in the Department of Social Anthropology, University of Cape Town, June 1992; Boonzaier, E.and Sharp, J., 1994, 'Ethnic Identity and Performance: Lessons from Namaqualand', *Journal of Southern Afri-can Studies*, 20(3): 405–15; Rasool, C. 1999. 'Cultural Performance and Fictions in Identity: the Case of the Khoisan of the Southern Kalahari, 1936–1937', in Y. Dladla (ed.) *Voices, Values and Identities Symposium*; Sharp, J., and Douglas, S.,1996, 'Prisoners of their Reputation? The Veterans of the "Bushman" Battalions in South Africa', in P. Skotnes (ed.) *Miscast: Negotiating the Presence of the Bushmen*; White, H., 1995, *In the Tradition of the Forefathers: Bushman traditionality at Kagga Kamma*.

towards cultural struggles and ethnic mobilisation strategies, which were regarded as playing into the hands of apartheid divide and rule policies. From the perspective of many Left intellectuals in the universities,[7] labour unions, and political organisations such as Unity Movement, the South African Communist Party (SACP), Pan Africanist Congress (PAC) and the African National Congress (ANC), ethnicity and 'tribalism' (Mafeje 1971) constituted forms of false consciousness promoted and abetted by Pretoria's architects of the homelands and Separate Development policies. The end of apartheid, along with the retreat of socialism and class-based mass mobilisation, meant that there was virtually no opposition from the Left, or from the state for that matter, to the cultural struggles of San people in South Africa. In fact, ethnicity and race had come to replace class as the keywords of the new official political discourse. Neither was there significant state opposition towards SASI's intimate involvement with international donors, NGOs and indigenous organisations that actively promoted self-determination and cultural rights for indigenous peoples. It was within this dramatically changed political landscape that indigenous Nama, San and Griqua ethnic revitalisation movements took place.[8]

The politics of authenticity: the 'real thing' or just 'faking it'

Non-Aboriginal Australians enjoy ancient traditions while suspecting the authenticity of the Aboriginal subject. Aboriginal Australians enjoy their traditions while suspecting the authenticity of themselves. (Povinelli 1999a)

On 1st July 1999, only a few months after the land signing agreement, Roger Friedman and Benny Gool reported in the *Cape Times* that 'fake bushmen' were being employed at the internationally renowned bushman tourist village at Kagga Kamma Nature Reserve.[9] In an article entitled, 'Fake San on Show: The great bushman tourist scam' (*Cape Times*, 1 July 1999), Friedman accused the Kagga Kamma management of 'passing off non-bushmen as the "genuine article" for the gratification of tourists'.[10] What also emerged from the article was a deepening schism between western and traditional bushmen at the new San resettlement

---

7 See Magubane, B., 1973, 'The Xhosa in town revisited: Urban social anthropology – A failure in method and theory', *American Anthropologist*, 75: 1701-14; Mafeje, A., 1971, 'Ideology of tribalism', *Journal of Modern African Studies*, 4(2); Boonzaier, E., and Sharp, J.S. (eds.) 1988, *South African Keywords: the uses and abuses of political concepts*.

8 The concept 'ethnic revitalisation' first appeared in Wallace, A., 1956, 'Revitalization Movements'. *American Anthropologist*, 58: 264–81. Elsewhere I have discussed problems with similar concepts such as Eric Hobsbawm and T.O. Ranger's 'invented tradition' and Emile Boonzaier and John Sharp's 'staged ethnicity'. For the purposes of this chapter I will use Wallace's concept to refer to self-conscious cultural constructions and strategies of ethnogenesis that, while often deployed for instrumental ends such as gaining access to land and state and donor resources, can at the same time be an attempt to reconstitute 'community' and cultural memories and identities following historical experiences of genocide, colonialism, and land and cultural dispossession. These concepts also need to take into account that it is often powerful outsiders (e.g., donors, NGOs, filmmakers, academics, state officials) who do the naming and who shape the parameters within which these identity constructions take place.

9 For an excellent ethnographic study of 'bushman tourism' at Kagga Kamma see White, H., 1995, *In the Tradition of the Forefathers: Bushman Traditionality at Kagga Kamma*.

10 *Cape Times*, 1 July 1999.

adjacent to the KGNP. I too had heard NGO workers and community members refer to the growing western/traditional bushmen divide during my visits to the Kalahari in early 1999.

The 'Great bushman tourist scam' uncovered by Friedman and Gool took place only a few months after the successful conclusion of the land claim. Following the handover ceremony, the ≠khomani San had decided to leave Kagga Kamma and settle at Welkom, a small settlement adjacent to the Park. After a decade of involvement in bushman tourism at Kagga Kamma they planned to establish their own tourism initiatives at their newly acquired farms. In response to the departure of the bushmen, the Kagga Kamma management had brought in a number of new bushmen who, according to Friedman and Gool, were in reality Coloureds from neighbouring farms. Isak Kruiper, the ex-leader of the Kagga Kamma group and traditional head of the ≠khomani San, told the *Cape Times* that it was 'very hurtful that the owner of Kagga Kamma is continuing to display bushmen [even though] they are not there. .. Kagga Kamma must close down or be honest with tourists and tell them that the people are Coloured'.[11] While, the Kagga Kamma tour guide had initially told the *Cape Times* reporter that they had '100% pure bushmen', the owner, Heinrich de Waal, later conceded that he had offered employment to Coloured farm workers, some of whom were married to bushmen. According to de Waal, although it was not ethical to tell people they are bushmen, 'there is no such thing as a "100% bushman"'. He justified the employment of Coloured people on the grounds that the Kruiper family had left Kagga Kamma and they urgently needed to keep the bushman business running. Friedman also solicited the views of members of SASI in his quest to get to the bottom of the Kagga Kamma scandal. SASI's director accused the Kagga Kamma management of violating fair trade agreements in their use of 'fake bushmen', and Chennels stated that Kagga Kamma's use of 'pretend bushmen' was insulting to both the San and the public. However, during my numerous conversations and interviews with Chennels it became clear that he recognised the difficulties and inconsistencies that surfaced when attempting to define the exact boundaries of the ≠khomani community. In fact, he pointed out that even the term '≠khomani San' was being questioned in the light of recent linguistic and historical research.

This concern with bushman authenticity is an age-old preoccupation that goes back to the first arrival of Europeans on African soil. The problem of classifying 'bushmen' created considerable anxiety amongst European travelers, scholars and administrators. Attempts to resolve this problem have generally taken the form of scientific inquiry into whether these people are 'pure products', fakes or hybrids. Language, genealogies, bodily features and livelihood strategies have gone into such classificatory exercises. However, the cultural hybridity of 'bushmen' has posed enormous problems for those seeking neat and unambiguous classifications. One of the responses to such classificatory quagmires has been the anxious repetition of bushman stereotypes. Such stereotypes continue to frame images of bushmen in popular culture, museum dioramas and tourist spectacles at Kagga Kamma and the San settlement near KGNP.

[11] Ibid.

The colonial stereotype of the pure and pristine bushman hunter and gatherer has also been embraced and articulated from below. Members of the Kruiper clan,[12] for example, appear to have strategically deployed bushman stereotypes in order to draw a clear line between themselves as traditionalists and the westernised bushmen in their midst.[13] This representational strategy feeds international donor conceptions of 'bushman' authenticity and it is likely to continue to influence San struggles over access to scarce resources such as land, traditional leadership and donor funding. It is also being used as claimants are being called upon to define the exact boundaries of the beneficiary community at their new settlement area.

Whereas some donors, fly-by-night consultants and tourists may view the ≠khomani San as the 'pure product', as pristine hunter gatherers, NGO fieldworkers and consultants such as Roger Chennels and Nigel Crawhall[14] of SASI have a far more nuanced and complex understanding of this community. Chennels' direct interactions with the San over a period of more than a decade has allowed him to recognise the ambiguities, hybridities and contradictions of San identities and local constructions of tradition and community. Although as their lawyer he recognised that the land claim process required coherent and consistent narratives of cultural continuity and belonging,[15] Chennels and the San now have to grapple with the problem of competing claims on who is ≠khomani San and who is not. These are realpolitik and pragmatic questions that will determine who may or may not join the ≠khomani San Communal Property Association (CPA) and gain access to land and state resources. Chennels expects the boundaries of the ≠khomani San community to remain unstable and highly contested, and openly acknowledges the fraught nature and fragility of current attempts at creating a sense of community (personal communication). He also recognises the troubling implications of these problems for the development of viable livelihood strategies at the new San settlements. Chennels' intermediary position as a cultural broker between the San claimant community and the donors becomes apparent when he points to the difficulty of explaining this complexity to funders. Whereas donors expect to find 'real bushmen' when they visit the Kalahari, Chennels is aware that many San claimants have in the past seen themselves as Coloureds rather than the descendants of San hunter-gatherers:

> [They are now] landowners with 40,000 hectares of farming land, and 25,000 hectares of game reserve. They'll have to train people to do the tracking and all those things to fill that space. But probably the most major challenge is trying to make the myth that we've actually created in order to win the land claim now become a reality. It is the myth that there is a

[12] The Kruiper clan is a term that is widely used to refer to David Kruiper and his network of kin and supporters. They are often perceived to be the original land claimants.

[13] *Cape Times*, 1 July 1999.

[14] Nigel Crawhall, a socio-linguist, has been instrumental in identifying the few remaining ≠khomani San-speakers in the Northern Cape Province. Along with the anthropologist and filmmaker Hugh Brody, Crawhall is currently involved in the audio-visual documentation of the language and life histories of these San speakers. Crawhall and Brody believe that these language projects, oral histories and accounts of San cultural practices are invaluable local resources that can translate into social capital. They can also function as inter-generational sources of cultural transmission and thereby contribute towards social cohesion and community solidarity.

[15] For a discussion on land claims and indigenous identities see Robins, S. 2000. 'Land Struggles and the Politics and Ethics of Representing "Bushman" History and Identity', *Kronos: Journal of Cape History, University of Western Cape*, 26: 56–75.

community of ≠khomani San. At the moment there is no such thing. It's a group of relations who are in the Northern Cape diaspora, and Dawid Kruiper is their symbolic leader ... Many of them know that he is responsible, that's why he's got his leadership position ... He stepped into a gap where there was no one before, and no one is fighting for that space. He has created the title, the traditional leader of the ≠khomani, and no one else challenges him ... SASI's job is to actually help their lives become more meaningful, and there's a need for it. We have to try and find a way of helping the ≠khomani understand what it means to be ≠khomani. Do they give jobs only to ≠khomani people? Do they have affirmative action for ≠khomani in a ≠khomani homeland? Do they call it a homeland, a cultural homeland? How will they perceive themselves, as a tribe or a people? I think SASI's role is very much about culture and development, around the cultural imperative of actually creating a community. Because there's a landowner, a legal entity, which has not yet really been filled, it's a potential entity at this moment. *So that is quite a difficult thing to tell the funders, to explain that some of the people who come to the meetings and to the elections have not actually seen a San themselves.* They are actually curious. They know their grandparents spoke this language or were of San, so they have this potential affinity. They're almost like members coming to a club not quite sure whether to join. They're only going to join the club if we make it meaningful for them to join, in a way that does not threaten their 'civilised' status. That I find is the real challenge. (Interview with Roger Chennels of SASI; my italics)

Whereas the original claimant community comprised 350 adults, the current numbers of the ≠khomani San community are estimated to be close to 1,000 adults spread over the Mier area in the Northern Cape, Botswana and Namibia (Roger Chennels, 1999, personal communication). With the growing awareness of the development and income-generation possibilities of the R15 million land claim settlement, it is to be expected that the numbers could increase further. It is as yet unclear what rules of inclusion and exclusion will be used to define rights to membership and access to ≠khomani San resources. Ultimately it will be up to the ≠khomani San leadership to come up with the criteria for membership of the CPA. In addition, the CPA will have to develop the capacity to make decisions concerning natural resource management and so on. During 1999, however, it became clear that there were tensions between the decision-making procedures stipulated in the CPA Constitution and the ad hoc decisions of the traditional leadership, for instance Dawid Kruiper's decision to shoot springbok on one of the farms.

Subsequent to the land signing ceremony, tensions intensified between the 'traditionalists' under Dawid Kruiper and the so-called western bushmen under the CPA leader Petrus Vaalbooi.[16] The traditionalists called for the severance of ties with their westernised relatives under the leadership of Petrus Vaalbooi, the son of Elsie Vaalbooi, one of the handful of ≠khomani San-speakers alive at the time of the land claim.[17] They even went as far as calling for the division of the San land claim area into two sections: the westernised stock farmers of the Vaalbooi group could have the farms outside the Park, and the traditionalist Kruiper clan would take the 25 000 hectares inside the Park.[18] The following section discusses how

---

[16] *Cape Times*, 16 September 1999.

[17] It was this split in the community that led Dawid Kruiper to make the following press statement: 'The traditional people say I must share 50/50 with Vaalie [Petrus Vaalbooi] or he would end up controlling all our land. I have told our lawyer it must be like that. We must divide the land to achieve peace between the San Association and the traditionalists' (*Cape Times*, 16 September 1999).

[18] Ibid.

this divide was itself largely a product of the dual mandate of donors and NGOs that wished both to preserve San tradition *and* to inculcate Western ideas about civil society and democratic accountability.

The politics of tradition and leadership in the Kalahari

The divergent leadership styles of the key players at KGNP heightened the divide between the traditionalists and the westerners. Petrus Vaalbooi, the former chair-person of the ≠khomani San CPA, is an eloquent and savvy political player. He cuts an impressive figure in national and international indigenous peoples conference circles. Vaalbooi is just as comfortable making polite conversation with President Thabo Mbeki or negotiating with the ministers of constitutional development and land affairs, as he is occupying the centre stage at UN indigenous peoples forums in Geneva. Vaalbooi's political style contrasts dramatically with the more low pro-file and parochial traditional leader, Dawid Kruiper. Moreover, whereas Vaalbooi is a relatively competent participant in development and bureaucratic discourses, Kruiper is not able to engage nearly as effectively in these discursive arenas. In addition, while Vaalbooi has commercial livestock interests, Kruiper is perceived to be only concerned with 'the bush', cultural tourism and hunting and gathering.

The responses of various donors, NGOs and academics to these diametrically opposed leadership practices and life-style orientations contributed towards exac-erbating this divide. For example, whereas members of SASI supported Kruiper's attempts to establish 'traditional' and culturally authentic activities such as craft production, bush knowledge and animal-tracking skills as part of eco-tourism proj-ects, those NGOs concerned with rural development tended to support Vaalbooi and the western bushmen who were involved in commercial livestock production. The involvement of Khoisan activists in the question of traditional leadership rein-forced these lines of division.[19] The tension between democratic decision-making processes promoted by the CPA Constitution and the centralised and personalised character of traditional leadership seemed extremely difficult to resolve. These contradictory objectives, I argue, lie at the heart of indigenous peoples NGOs' unstated, and perhaps unintentional, dual mandate: to promote the cultural sur-vival of indigenous peoples and their traditional institutions, and to socialise them into becoming modern citizens within a global civil society. These NGOs often seek to promote both cultural authenticity and democratic accountability in their engagements with indigenous peoples.

The traditionalist leadership continues to draw on dress and language as power-

[19] These problems raise ethical dilemmas as to whether NGOs or the state have the right or obligation to intervene in the institutional arrangements and decision-making processes of the ≠khomani San. It could be argued that outsider intervention is problematic given the San's historical experience of paternalistic rela-tions with a range of outsiders, including white farmers, tourists, philanthropists, anthropologists, NGOs and the state. Yet it is equally plausible to argue that not to intervene simply reinforces already existing divisions in ways that strengthen patriarchal institutions and further marginalise women. Whereas donors based in Europe and North America can continue to imagine the ≠khomani San as the living embodiment of har-monious hunter gatherer culture, Roger Chennels and SASI have had to continually engage with everyday social realities that throw up the dilemmas of intervening in differentiated and divided social groupings.

ful signs of authenticity and belonging in the Kalahari. For instance, the Kruiper traditionalists attempted to banish bushmen from entering the Witdraai settlement unless they wore the traditional skins or *!xai*. The handful of elderly San-speakers at Witdraai have also become the embodiment of authentic San identity, and they are regularly appropriated by competing groupings in divisive power struggles and public displays of authenticity. The three San-speaking Swartkop sisters, /Abaka Rooi, Keis Brow, /Una Rooi, for example, were often appropriated by various members of the ≠khomani community as embodied signs and custodians of San tradition. These particular processes of cultural appropriation were also made possible by SASI's concentration on San language projects.

This focus on language has also led to a situation whereby Afrikaans-speaking, western-dressed livestock farmers such as Petrus Vaalbooi and his brother have come to be seen as westernised bushmen, the 'impure product'. Dawid Kruiper has also become a victim of this process since he only speaks Nama and Afrikaans. Fluency in a San language, along with 'bush knowledge' and a history of employment and residence in the Park, has become a crucial marker of San identity. It has also had a powerful influence on local community politics. Whereas Kruiper's legitimacy as a traditional leader owed much to his claims that he was raised in the Park and learnt bush knowledge from his late father, Regopstaan Kruiper, this narrative was challenged by some San-speaking elders who claimed that the Nama and Afrikaans-speaking Kruiper was in Botswana at the time of the forced removals. These badges of authenticity and legitimacy continue to haunt San leaders and divide the community.

For San leaders like the Afrikaans-speaking Petrus Vaalbooi, who do not have direct access to these cultural markers, alternative legitimising strategies have to be deployed. Vaalbooi's rise to prominence as the first ≠khomani San Communal Property Association (CPA) chairperson was largely a result of his ability to engage with development and bureaucratic discourses. Vaalbooi's strength as a leader was also due to his ability as a translator and mediator of local San issues to broader national and international audiences. It is precisely these Western-style discursive competencies that are recognised and rewarded by NGOs and donors committed to promoting the values and democratic practices of civil society. At the same time, Vaalbooi's local legitimacy was built upon the fact that he is the son of the 97-year-old Elsie Vaalbooi, one of a dozen known ≠khomani San-speakers in South Africa. However, Vaalbooi's Achilles Heel was his inability to speak Nama or San, as well as his initial refusal to wear loincloths. The Afrikaans-speaking western-dressed Vaalbooi did not conform to popular notions of cultural authenticity embodied in the image of the primordial bushman. By 2005, however, Petrus Vaalbooi had taken to wearing traditional loincloths at important public events, for instance the signing of the *Hoodia* deal.[20]

While NGOs and donors tend to valorise these signs of authentic San culture – language, clothes and bodily vernacular – they also value individuals like Vaalbooi who are able to master development and governance discourses, and who

[20] Vaalbooi appears in traditional loincloths in Rehad Desai's documentary on *Hoodia* entitled, *Bushmen's Secret.*

appear to be willing to embrace the virtues of democratic accountability promoted by global civil society. The ambiguities of this dual mandate – of promoting of San cultural survival and the values and virtues of 'civil society' such democratic decision-making within the CPA – invoked a repetition of stereotypes about 'pure' and 'detribalised' bushmen that contributed towards the reinscription of an artificial divide between traditionalist and western bushmen.

Hybrid discourses and indigenous modernities in the Kalahari

Despite considerable evidence of the hybrid character of both NGOs' discourses and the everyday practices and identities of the San themselves, advocates of modernisation and traditionalism seem to share a common discomfort with the idea of the hybrid. Modernisers and traditionalists alike seem to believe in the necessity for pure categories and identities. However, the attempts to constitute a purified San tradition in the Kalahari created problems for traditionalists who found themselves unable to completely fit their own criteria and conceptions of authentic and pure San tradition. After all, most of them are Afrikaans- and Nama-speaking former farm workers or National Parks employees with extremely tenuous ties to a hunter-gatherer existence. However, the more porous and precarious these claims on authentic San identity and tradition, the more intense struggles to eradicate the influence of exogenous forces of modernity can become. Even the most fervent San traditionalists were deeply implicated in the discursive webs of modernity. This situation, it would seem, is largely a product of historical encounters with the West, including colonialism, Christianity, capitalist wage labour, the state, donors, NGOs, academics, journalists, white farmers, tourists and so on. Despite the efforts of outsiders, and the San themselves, to create the myth of the 'pure bushman', there was no escape from this hybrid condition that characterises the everyday social realities of the ≠khomani San.

It is perhaps paradoxical that the survival of San hunter and gatherer traditions has required that the traditionalists expend considerable energy accessing exogenous modern means of production, cultural tourism, wage labour, and government and donor grants, for example. As Marshall Sahlins (1999) notes, 'the survival of indigenous peoples such as hunter-gatherers is often not a result of their isolation, but rather their subsistence is dependent on modern means of production, transportation and communication – rifles, snowmachines, motorised vessels and, at least in North America, CB radios and all-terrain vehicles – which they buy using money they have acquired from a variety of sources including public transfer payments, resource loyalties, wage labor and commercial fishing' (ibid.: 140)[21] Sahlins' comments suggest that these peoples need to engage with modern means of production but that this does not mean that they are simply swallowed up in the homogenising forces of modernity and globalisation. Instead, many of these

---

[21] Sahlins also writes: '"Develop-man" is the neo-Malanesian term for development; and it would not be wrong to repidginize it back to English as "the development of man", since the project it refers to is the use of foreign wealth in the expansion of feasting, politicking, subsidizing kinship, and other activities that make up the local conception of a human existence' (ibid.: ix).

groups adapt and recast their dependencies on modern means of production in order to reconstitute and reproduce their own cultural ideas and practices (ibid.). Similarly, by participating in NGO and donor-driven projects, indigenous groups such as the Kalahari San are drawing on the modern institutions and resources of a global civil society to reconstitute themselves as a traditional community. Indeed, it is precisely by invoking this dichotomy that traditionalists are able to ground an extremely unstable and hybrid San identity.

Sahlins and others refer to the integration of industrial technologies in indigenous sociologies and cosmologies as indigenous modernities. However, the pervasiveness of a western dichotomy of tradition and modernity continues to obscure the reality of localised processes that Sahlins describes as the indigenisation of modernity. Instead, of recognising this hybridisation, 'western' binary thinking contributes towards the persistent reassertion of an artificial divide between tradition and modernity. As will become evident in the following section, the construction of a dichotomy between San traditionalists and western bushmen in the Kalahari was, it would appear, itself partly a response to the contradictory demands of donors and NGOs for the San to simultaneously constitute themselves both as Late Stone Age survivors and modern citizens of the nation state.

Mixed messages and crossed lines?: 'cultural survival' and the 'civilising mission'

Elsewhere I have written about the ways in which the land claims process has contributed towards post-apartheid reclamations of Nama and San cultural identity (Robins 1997, 2000). Land claims in the Northern Cape, like elsewhere in the country, have become a catalyst for processes of ethnogenesis (Sharp 1996; Wilmsen and McAllister 1996) that reproduce apartheid-like ethnic categories and essentialist discourses. These ethnic categories and tribal discourses, however, are not simply imposed 'from above' by the state, donors or NGOs, but are also reinvented and reappropriated by land claimants themselves (Robins 2000). The following pages analyse NGOs as 'third parties', as inter-hierarchical brokers or mediators of state and donor discourses and agendas, as well as local community interests. Examining the ambiguous and intermediary structural and discursive location of SASI, and its involvement in the San land claim, can throw light on the complex and contradictory nature of the cultural politics of land, community, development and identity amongst the ≠khomani San people. It can also reveal the impact at the local level of the mixed messages of donor and NGO programmes.

Given that donors and NGOs tend to view indigenous peoples as both 'First People' and modern citizens-in-the-making, it is not surprising that SASI has sought to develop ways of combining charismatic and patriarchal styles of traditional leadership with the establishment of a ≠khomani San Communal Property Association (CPA), along with a Constitution and executive committee to ensure democratic procedures of accountability and decision-making. However, it soon became apparent that there was tension between the followers of 'western bushmen' under the then CPA chairperson, Petrus Vaalbooi, and San traditionalists under Dawid Kruiper.

It was during the post-settlement phase that rural development NGOs such as *Farm Africa* began to move into the Kalahari in order to assist the San to develop organisational capacity to deal with the more mundane administrative and development matters relating to land-use and livestock management. While SASI's decision to concentrate on First People status may have made strategic sense during the land claims process, this emphasis was perceived to be inadequate during the post-settlement phase.

In recent years NGOs have come to be seen by policy makers, development practitioners, donors, politicians and social scientists as conduits for the dissemination of western forms of liberalism, rights, citizenship, civil society and so on. Scholars of international relations have examined the impact of NGO coalitions and networks on international politics and their role in the formation of a post-Cold War international civil society (Fisher 1997). A key question here has been the problematic relationship between globally connected NGOs and the nation state. NGOs have also come to be seen as the most effective brokers and mediators of global discourses of Western liberal democracy and modernisation in the Third World. William Fisher (1997: 444) notes that NGOs have also been identified by advocates of neoliberalism as effective institutions for transferring training and skills that 'assist individuals and communities to compete in markets, to provide welfare services to those who are marginalised by the market, and to contribute to democratisation and the growth of a robust civil society, all of which are considered critical to the success of neoliberal economic policies'.[22] It would appear from all this interest in NGOs that they are indeed perceived to be the panacea for the promotion of liberal democracy and 'development' in the Third World.

This identification of NGOs as custodians and promoters of the virtues of liberal democracy has, however, been brought into question by the observation that, given the limited financial resources available, NGOs are becoming increasingly unaccountable and dependent on the whims and fancies of international donors, state aid agencies and corporate patrons. This has led some radical critics such as Petras and Veltmeyer (2001) and Hardt and Negri (2000) to accuse NGOs of being anti-democratic handmaidens of neoliberalism and global capital (see Chapter 1). Notwithstanding these critiques, NGOs continue to be lauded for promoting democratisation and the expansion of the core values of civil society (Fisher 1997: 444).

Recent studies of NGOs by William Fisher (ibid.), Elizabeth Garland (1999) and Steve Sampson (1996), as well as the emergence of a growing anthropological literature on the discourses of the development industry (for example, Cooper and Packard 1997; Crush 1995; Escobar 1995; Esteva 1992; Ferguson 1990), have raised important questions concerning the discursive construction of devel-

---

[22] Ibid. p. 444. According to Fisher (1997: 439–64), NGOs are praised by advocates of modernisation and liberal democracy, and radicals who view NGOs as catalysts for social movements that promote popular democratic alternatives to development. While it is clear from the above that NGOs mean different things to different folk, there is a widespread tendency to homogenise this extremely heterogeneous category of institutions.

opment 'problems', 'solutions' and 'target populations'. James Ferguson's 1990 *Anti-Politics Machine*, for instance, draws attention to the problematic ways in which development discourses produce homogenous target populations such as 'less developed countries' (LDCs), 'the Third World', female-headed households, and 'traditional farmers'. The San too have been constructed as a target population by a range of social actors and institutions, including the state, donors and NGOs. Geneva-based donors, indigenous rights organisations and NGOs may conceive of the San as a uniform and homogenous 'target category' of pristine hunter gatherers, but the closer one gets to the ground the more unstable, messy and differentiated this category begins to appear.

The view from below can be equally confusing. For example, whereas close-up observations of the Kalahari San might seem to suggest that they are totally captured within the everyday Western *habitus* of liberal development workers, teachers, missionaries, New Agers, and government bureaucrats, this intimate exposure to the 'civilising mission' does not necessarily mean that they seamlessly reproduce Western liberal political ideals and practices (see Garland 1999). The San 'target population' is a 'moving target', unable and unwilling to live up to either western fantasies of the bushmen as Late Stone Age survivors, or developmentalist visions of the San as normalised, disciplined and 'civilised' modern subjects ready to be recruited into an increasingly global civil society.

Elsewhere I have discussed various possible explanations for the tenacity of popular perceptions of the ≠khomani San as 'First People', as the living embodiments of Late Stone Age hunter-gatherers (see Robins 2000). It is by now hardly news to note that these tenacious primordialist fantasies emanate from a variety of sources including anthropologists, filmmakers, museum curators, donors, NGOs, journalists, tourists and so on. The following section investigates the specific ways in which such notions are reproduced, challenged and reconfigured in the context of the ≠khomani San land claim. This will involve an analysis of the disjunctures, ambiguities and contradictions embedded in discourses on indigenous peoples that are disseminated by bodies such as the United Nations Working Group for Indigenous Peoples (UNWGIP) and international donors. It will also involve an analysis of how these global discourses are understood and reconfigured by the ≠khomani San community and by SASI[23] given the prevailing socio-economic and political realities in San settlements adjacent to the Kalahari Gemsbok National Park (KGNP).

---

[23] While having to engage with international discourses on indigenous peoples, SASI has also had to engage with the specificities of the South African context. This has led to a critical engagement with global indigenous rights discourse and raised important questions that interrogate some of the assumptions embedded in these discourses. While SASI made a valuable contribution in preparing the San claimant community for a successful land claim, the chapter raises questions concerning the possible relations of dependency between NGOs and international donor organisations. In what ways does SASI's relationship with its overseas donors influence its development strategies? Can this relationship in any way account for the apparent prioritising of cultural and language projects rather than rural development interventions that address the more mundane conditions of rural poverty and social fragmentation that continue to characterise everyday life at the Kalahari San settlement? These difficult questions are raised in order to contribute towards critical and reflexive development practices that facilitate social transformation and upliftment amongst marginalised people in the Northern Cape and elsewhere.

Citizens and bushmen: discourses on indigenous identity

In South Africa there are a number of groups currently claiming indigenous status in terms of the internationally recognised (UNWGIP) use of the term. These would include the Nama (Xhoi or Khoekhoe),[24] San, Griqua and !Korrana.[25] The San, Nama and Griqua were classified as Coloured in terms of the 1955 race classification legislation introduced by the Nationalist Government that came into power in 1948.[26] This legislation was accompanied by vigorous state-led assimilation policies. For example, Nama children were forced to use Afrikaans in school, and an Afrikaans, Christian, Coloured identity was imposed upon the Nama through the institutions of church and state. Many people with San, Nama and Griqua ancestry also opted to identify with this Coloured identity due to the negative connotations and racist discrimination associated with the terms 'hottentot' and 'boesman' under colonialism and apartheid. As a result, the San and Nama languages and culture have almost disappeared. Whereas Nama is still spoken in the Northern Cape Province in northern parts of Namaqualand such as Richtersveld, it has virtually vanished in the more missionised southern Namaqualand settlements such Leliefontein (Robins 1997). Unlike Nama/Coloureds and black Africans, San people were not given their own Reserves as it was assumed that they were 'extinct' or thoroughly assimilated into the Coloured population. This has also contributed towards the particularly marginalised character of San identity. This marginalisation is evident in the fact that there are only approximately a dozen identified ≠khomani San speakers throughout South Africa.

The response of the ANC government to the dramatic reclamations of Nama, San and Griqua identity that began the early 1990s, has been one of caution and ambivalence. The government remains wary of an indigenous rights movement that could become a vehicle for exclusivist ethnic politics. This deep-standing distrust of ethnic politics probably also comes out of a historical legacy of apartheid and rightwing Afrikaner nationalism, as well as the bloody clashes between the Inkatha Freedom Party (IFP) and ANC supporters in KwaZulu-Natal and Gauteng. It would also appear that the ANC, as an unambiguously modernist organisation, is concerned that an accommodation of communitarianism could end up contradicting the underlying principles of liberal democracy.[27] From a more pragmatic

---

[24] Nama is the only surviving Khoe language in South Africa.

[25] There are approximately five to ten thousand Nama-speaking people in the Northern Cape mostly concentrated in the northern Namaqualand area, along the Orange River.

[26] There are some 3,600,000 South Africans who identify themselves as 'Coloured' (*Statistics SA*, 1998: section 2.5). The category of 'Coloured' disguises the cultural heterogeneity of people many of whom have European, African, Khoe, San, Indian, Indonesian, Malay and slave backgrounds. The majority of so-called Coloureds do not identify themselves as indigenous Khoe or San. However, the gains made by a growing indigenous rights movement could encourage many of these people to reclaim and recognise African, San and Khoe ancestry, which has tended to be suppressed in favour of a stress on their European and Christian background.

[27] The hesitance on the part of the South African government to take on international definitions and conventions on indigenous rights also stems from a belief that South Africa has specific and unique circumstances that have to be addressed. These specificities, it is argued, militate against the uncritical embrace of international conventions and legal policies on indigenous people. Johan Meiring, a state

position, the enormous logistical difficulties experienced in attempting to process the thousands of land claims already submitted to the Land Claims Court may have contributed towards the government's reluctance to encourage indigenous groups to agitate for aboriginal land title along the lines of Australia and New Zealand land law.

The official usage of the term 'indigenous' in South Africa has come to mean something different to the way it is used by international donors, the United Nations and various indigenous peoples forums and activist groups. Although there is as yet no clearly stated definition of the term, it appears twice in the South African Constitution (Chapters 6 and 26). The Constitution's use of the term in fact derives from the common South African use of the word 'indigenous' to refer to the languages and legal customs of the African majority of Bantu-language speakers.[28] In South Africa, like other parts of southern Africa, the term 'indigenous' is used to distinguish the black African majority from the European settlers and Asian minorities. It seldom refers to the notion of First Peoples.

Khoi and San advocates and activists are critical of the government's failure to adopt international indigenous rights (First Peoples) legal frameworks. For instance, SASI linguist and development consultant Nigel Crawhall believes the South African government's rights-based paradigm 'ignores the inability of marginalised indigenous communities to effectively hold the state accountable for implementation of its rights'. It is with this in mind that Crawhall continues to call for the specific recognition of 'Indigenous Africans', in line with international conceptions of First Peoples.

The common use of the term 'indigenous' in South Africa refers to the Khoi and San as well as the Bantu-speaking majority. This is somewhat different to UNWGIP's use of the term to refer to minority First Peoples of aboriginal descent and with distinct territorial and cultural identities. The ANC government's apparent reluctance to take on board this UN definition is a consequence of its belief that the majority of black Africans and Coloureds are indigenous South Africans.[29] For instance, when asked by a journalist whether the successful resolution of the ≠khomani San land claim represented the government's intention to recognise Khoi and San as 'First People', former minister of land affairs, Derek Hanekom, flatly refuted this assumption. He claimed that virtually all black South Africans

---

[27 ctnd] ethnologist in the Department of Constitutional Development, echoed this view. Meiring told me in an interview in Pretoria that his department's position was that 'we should really understand the African, South African, situation of these people very well before we can just accept international definitions [of indigenous rights] or even the Convention itself.' I encountered similar caution in my interview with Johan Beukman, a senior official in the Department of Constitutional Development. Beukman drew attention to potential problems that could arise in simply recognising traditional authority amongst the San. Although Dawid Kruiper is recognised as the ≠khomani San traditional leader this is an unofficial designation. Meanwhile vocal Griqua and other 'Khoisan' leaders were vigorously calling for official recognition in the house of traditional leaders. Beukman's Department responded by establishing a commission to investigate Nama, San and Griqua political leadership structures.

[28] 76.7% of South Africans are considered to be African (i.e., of Bantu-language-speaking origin). Whites of European descent comprise 10.9%; Coloureds are 8.9% and Indians 2.6% (*Statistics SA*, 1998).

[29] The term 'Black' is often used to refer specifically to black Africans who speak Bantu languages. It is also used more broadly to refer to Indians, Coloureds, Khoi, San and Africans, i.e., 'non-whites'. The term 'Black', like 'African' and 'Coloured', is a highly unstable and contested term.

had suffered under colonialism and apartheid and it would not make sense to separate out and privilege the experiences of one group on the basis of claims to autochthonous, aboriginal or First Peoples status. As Hanekom pointed out, the land claims cut-off date is in any case 1913, which rules out claims to aboriginal land rights. From the ANC's perspective, redress has to address the needs of all South African citizens disadvantaged by racial legislation.[30]

San and Khoisan activists believe that the constitution ought to recognise the very specific conditions of marginalisation of the San and Nama in South Africa. They argue that this exceptionality is evident in the observation that there are only about a dozen known ≠khomani San-speakers left in South Africa.[31] This alone, they argue, makes the San one of the most vulnerable and marginalised groups in South Africa. The ANC, like other African governments, disagrees, and has refused to accept United Nations declarations on indigenous peoples.

The ANC is clearly unwilling to encourage an indigenous rights movement that would challenge the 1913 Land Act cut-off date for the recognition of land claims. In terms of the current Land Restitution Act 22 of 1994 only racially based land dispossession from 1913 to 1994 is recognised. Some San and Khoi activists have demanded that the Act should allow for indigenous land claims going back hundreds of years. In addition, since it was founded in 1913, the ANC has embraced a Western-style liberal democratic and rights-based model which cannot easily accommodate communitarian political institutions such as African traditional leadership, which SASI and Khoisan and San activists are now also calling for. However, given the concessions granted to African traditional leaders in the recent past, including the establishment of a House of Traditional Leaders, the government is regularly reminded by Khoisan and San activists that it has already set a precedent. In fact, traditional leaders have recently been given more powers in terms of land rights in communal areas. This perhaps explains why, despite a reluctance to ratify international conventions on indigenous rights, the ANC government has nonetheless taken seriously the dire predicament of the ≠khomani and !Xu/Khwe San. Apart from the provision of land, the government has also initiated a process aimed at addressing the specific needs and cultural rights of San, Nama and Griqua communities, although it remains to be seen whether this will bear fruit.[32]

---

[30] The following excerpt from an interview with Roger Chennels illustrates the different meanings the term 'indigenous' has in South Africa compared to international forums such as the UNWGIP: 'When we talk about indigenous peoples in Geneva we are talking about a new [term] created by the United Nations and Native Americans and others who choose not to call themselves minorities ... The Decade of Indigenous Peoples refers to those people. Xhosas and Kikuyus are not part of it, they are majority people who participate in the mainstream politics of their countries. But this term is very problematic in Africa, and I can understand why South Africa, thinking of its [black] African responsibilities, can't just take the term on, because if they go to the OAU and start talking about indigenous peoples it could be very confusing ... So without enough understanding of the term it could become dangerous and difficult. I wouldn't actually fight too much about it [because] the term is going to remain confusing. The French meaning "indigene" just means related to the earth, the soil. We're all indigene in some way. I don't think that the ANC government is being backward or otherwise, they're just being very sensible.'

[31] There are about 4500 former Angolan Khwe and !Xu San now living near Kimberley.

[32] SASI has been a key player in promoting this indigenous rights agenda. Notwithstanding a reluctance to accept the UNWGIP definition of the term 'indigenous', the South African government has given the San and Nama significant resources, including land and state funds for indigenous language projects.

The question of strategic essentialism

Rather than focusing exclusively on chasing after constitutionally enshrined rights for indigenous people, SASI's lawyer, Roger Chennels, is also concerned with the enormous challenges of creating viable local community structures and livelihood strategies. It is here, at the more mundane and immediate level of everyday life – poverty, conflict and social fragmentation – that Chennels locates the San agenda. However, it is not only these material realities that need to be addressed. Chennels and Crawhall believe that tapping into San local knowledge and the historical narratives of elders could be a valuable source of social capital in the quest to forge a collective sense of belonging, psychological well-being and social cohesion, as well as facilitating the development of viable livelihood strategies. There need not be an artificial dichotomy between more materialist-based rural development strategies of NGOs such as Farm Africa, and SASI's cultural projects which are aimed at stimulating social capital formation through inter-generational knowledge transfer. However, it remains to be seen to what degree these indigenous knowledges and cultural practices can be used as a basis for cultural survival and economic sustainability for present and future generations of San.

Given the strong interest of international donors in the 'cultural survival' of vanishing cultures and languages, it could be argued that it still makes strategic sense for San communities, and SASI, to stress the importance of their hunter-gatherer lifestyle, indigenous knowledge and San cultural continuity. The deployment of these strategies to gain donor funding may also contribute towards reconstituting kinship and other activities that contribute towards the remaking of San conceptions of human existence. However, endorsing primordialist notions of the San as hunter-gatherers could also contribute towards the devaluation and marginalisation of alternative livelihood strategies and social practices that do not conform to this stereotypical bushman image. For instance, San livestock farmers are often perceived to be less authentically San by donors even though, for many ≠khomani San, goats and sheep have been, and continue to be, the most viable livelihood strategy in the arid Kalahari region. While livestock production is in fact taking place on the newly acquired farms, it has contributed towards growing tensions between so-called 'traditionalists' who claim to prefer the hunter gatherer/cultural tourism option, and livestock farmers who are referred to as the 'western bushmen'. As was mentioned earlier, the media, academics, NGOs and donors are not entirely innocent in these processes.

Anthropologists and historians have devoted enormous time and resources towards proving or disproving 'bushman authenticity'. This obsessive preoccupation with cultural authenticity is not of course limited to scholars. For example, when Donald Bain wanted to establish a Bushman reserve in South Africa in the 1930s he encountered strong opposition from white farmers who, fearing shortages

---

32 ctnd The prominence of references to the San in Mbeki's speeches and the use of San words in the new coat of arms are signs that the new state views 'the San' as a cultural asset and symbolic icon of the new nation. Despite these significant material and symbolic gestures, indigenous land and cultural rights are not recognized in South African law, and there are no indications that this is likely to change in the foreseeable future.

of farm labour, claimed that the reserve was unnecessary as there were no 'real bushmen' left. In recent years, 'bushman' tourism and the ≠khomani San land claim have once again triggered academic and popular interest in the perennial question of bushmen authenticity. More than fifty years after Bain's aborted attempt at salvaging bushman culture through the establishment of a reserve, the issue of bushmen authenticity remains as loaded as ever. It would appear that the bushmen have once again become the lightning rod for academic and media discourses on cultural difference and authenticity. It is as if they have come to represent the last repository of absolute alterity, as a mythic, primordial Other. Ironically, they have also become intellectual fodder for countless academic projects aimed at debunking 'bushman myths' and primordialist essentialism.

The perceived uniqueness of the Kalahari San and their land claim attracted enormous media, donor and NGO interest. It also captivated President Mbeki and the former minister of lands, Derek Hanekom, whose personal involvement in the claim played a particularly significant role in ensuring its success. It appears that the ANC government perceived the Kalahari land claim as a one-off opportunity to settle the potentially troubling question of pre-1913 indigenous land rights. In addition, popular images of the primordial bushman in the Kalahari not only fuel media and scholarly interest, but also shape government, NGO and donor perceptions and development strategies and priorities. For instance, San development projects are known to receive generous funding from international donor organisations for whom the Kalahari bushman represents the last of the surviving Late Stone Age hunter gatherers. Similarly, it could be argued that the R15 million San land claim 'jumped the queue' precisely because the San are perceived to be such a valuable political and tourist commodity by the state, NGOs, donors and the media. President Mbeki's African Renaissance, South Africa's quest for a permanent seat on the UN Security Council, and the race for votes in the Northern Cape probably all played a significant role in the ANC government's last minute rush to address San land and language rights in the run-up to the 1999 general elections. Another factor was the international visibility it provided to South Africa's shining human rights record. Although political opportunism alone cannot account for the whole story, it would appear that the San land claim was indeed perceived to be symbolically and politically strategic by the ANC government. This does not imply, however, that they were passive victims of the machinations of powerful political elites; after all, they managed to win back their land back and continue to secure access to state resources. Nor were they merely passive victims of the representations, political agendas and development discourses of powerful outsiders.

Representations of bushmen as First People that are reproduced daily at South African museum dioramas and San tourist villages continue to ignore the devastating consequences of San genocide, land and cultural dispossession and contemporary rural poverty and social fragmentation. However, drawing attention to this devastating San past and present does not necessarily appeal to tourists who want to see the Kruiper clan dressed in loincloths and carrying bows and arrows. Neither does it necessarily appeal to donors looking for First People. It would seem that Dawid Kruiper and his followers recognise that these 'traditional' bushman images can become crucial cultural and economic resources in their quest for a future that is more than mere cultural survival. They are creative and self-conscious producers of the cultural commodities that fuel a fledgling tourist and donor-driven economy. The investment of individuals in mastering this ≠khomani San history and identity also appears to be more than simply the instrumental manipulation of 'culture' in order to gain access to material resources. They are also cultural practices aimed at the recuperation of social memory and identity similar to other cultural reclamations taking place throughout post-apartheid South Africa.

The problem with such strategic essentialism, as Gayatri Spivak (1988) points out, is that it can end up obscuring intra-community differences along class, age or gender lines. These ethnic strategies of mobilisation also tend to ignore and degrade cultural hybridities in the name of pure essences and cultural continuity, thereby encouraging the kinds of tensions between pure and westernised bushmen that emerged in the Kalahari. Moreover, such an approach could render the San increasingly dependent on powerful donors and create obstacles for San communities seeking to develop independent and effective local community and leadership structures. It is also likely to alienate the ≠khomani San from their Coloured and Nama-speaking neighbours in Northern Cape. Growing divisions and tensions have in fact occurred between the claimant community and their communal farmer neighbours in the Mier area. This culminated in legal contestation of the San claim by Mier residents. The matter was eventually resolved through a negotiated settlement whereby Mier communal farmers also received state land and resources as compensation for land dispossession under apartheid. Nonetheless, instead of encouraging strategic ties with their neighbours, a donor focus on San exceptionalism and First People status could end up isolating and alienating this claimant community from potential political allies in the neighbouring communal areas and rural towns. An ethnic separatist strategy that was perceived to be strategic during the San land-claim process, and which was supported by NGOs and donors, could contribute towards erecting an artificial barrier between the ≠khomani San and neighbouring Coloured and Baster communities, even though many of the San claimants come from these neighbouring areas and have close kinship ties with people living there. A narrowly defined donor focus on indigenous San could create problematic socio-spatial and political divisions and inequalities amongst these culturally hybrid and impoverished rural people of the Northern Cape Province.[33]

Ethnic separatist strategies were initiated at the expense of the possibility of San participation in broad class-based social movements and development initiatives involving Coloured, black African and Nama communal farmers, farm workers, the unemployed and other marginalised groups in the Northern Cape region. However, given the fact that this political mobilisation is not taking place, and that it is unlikely to take place in the near future, it probably made strategic sense for the ≠khomani San, with the help of SASI, to concentrate on taking care

---

[3] See Kay Warren's 1998 *Indigenous Movements and their Critics: Pan Maya Activism in Guatemala*, p. 6, for a discussion of the arguments of critics who maintain that Pan-Mayan 'ethnic revitalization' poses a threat to national unity and political stability.

of their own needs and concerns. However, this approach confined the San to an 'ethnic cage'. SASI has not worked with non-San communities as this could both jeopardise its ability to tap into Northern doncr circuits earmarked specifically for indigenous people and could also spread the organisation's limited resources too thinly. Restricting their work to San issues probably also made sense given SASI's identification of the San as a hyper-marginalised community with very specific social and cultural needs and predicaments.

SASI could find itself in a situation where it is unable to entirely dismiss international donor desires for authentic First People, and yet unable to ignore the ambiguities, contradictions and messy social realities they encounter in their everyday encounters in the Kalahari. Chennels' comment on the difficulty of explaining this complexity to funders remains a troubling one. Meanwhile, recent developments in the Kalahari suggest that donors are uncertain whether they should fund cultural survival NGOs or more mainstream rural development NGOs. Some of the major donors have in fact recently provided significant support for rural development programmes at the Kalahari San settlement as a way of countering a perception, rightly or wrongly, that in the past the bulk of San donor resources went to cultural survival projects.

The following letter to the *Sunday Independent*, entitled 'Create lasting economic strategy for Nyae-Nyae', is a highly polemical attack on San cultural survival projects in Namibia. The writer, who claims to have spent 15 years at Nyae-Nyae, lambasts outsiders for promoting their own self-interested conceptions of bushman culture.[34] The letter was written in response to a prior article entitled 'Alcohol makes a desert of Namibians' hopes':[35]

> The people of Nyae-Nyae have their own culture just as all other people in Namibia have their own culture. This has nothing to do with the ability to keep animals and grow vegetables. The people of Bushmanland are perfectly capable of keeping cattle and growing vegetables. It might not be 'in their tradition', but neither was warfare nor alcohol. For 15 years I have witnessed NGOs, governments, trophy hunters, racketeers, conservationists, film makers, intellectuals and quasi-intellectuals and priests telling the people of Nyae-Nyae how they should preserve their 'culture' and run their lives. Culture and tradition can only survive if the people want it to. Paternalism from outsiders just won't do the trick. If anyone was really concerned about the wellbeing of the 'bushmen' of Nyae-Nyae, they would have created an economic environment diverse enough for the people to be able to feed themselves. This has not happened and never will as long as outsiders with their own agendas try to rule the roost.

The letter is an outright attack on what the author perceives to be the outside imposition of San cultural survival projects that do not adequately address San poverty and create viable livelihood options. There is a danger, however, that such blanket criticisms could be used to justify the imposition of rural development projects that fail to address adequately the specificities of the social and cultural aspects of everyday life in San communities. It could end up ignoring the valuable local knowledge and 'social capital' that SASI development consultants such as Nigel Crawhall and Roger Chennels believe is essential for any attempt to reconstitute

---

[34] *Sunday Independent*, 17 October 1999.
[35] *Sunday Independent*, 5 September 1999.

this highly fractured San community.

This indictment of outsider interventions could also end up failing to recognise the ways in which representations of San tradition and culture are fashioned from below by the San themselves. While the appropriation of essentialist notions of San cultural identity can contribute to the kinds of conflicts between traditionalist and western bushmen that occurred in the Kalahari, it is not inconceivable that these 'bushmen myths' could also contribute towards reconstituting the social fabric of community and revitalising local conceptions of San culture. Similarly, although San cultural politics could lead to forms of ethnic separatism and isolationism that undermine social and economic ties with non-San neighbours in adjacent communal areas and rural towns, there is no inevitability about this outcome. It would seem that San cultural politics does not have any pre-ordained script or teleology.

To break out of the ethnic mould of apartheid history, South African NGOs, and the San themselves, have to walk a fine line between negotiating the primordialist desires and fantasies of funders, and the need to gain access to development resources to empower poverty-stricken San communities. They will also need to negotiate the ambiguous and contradictory dual mandate of donors who seek to promote San 'cultural survival' while simultaneously inculcating the values and virtues of 'civil society' and liberal individualism, development and democracy. This could be a hard road to walk.

Conclusion

This chapter has focused on donors, NGOs and the San claimant community in its investigation of how the apparently contradictory agendas of San cultural survival and the promotion of the values and practices of civil society have impacted upon the ≠khomani San after the land claim. It is clear that the cultural politics of San identity, community and tradition is a highly complicated and shifting discursive field, and that the San are simultaneously enmeshed in donor and NGO projects of cultural recuperation and the 'civilising mission' of liberal democracy and the liberal modernist idea of the autonomous rights-bearing subject. It would also appear that, despite considerable evidence of the hybrid character of San local knowledges and everyday practices, the dual mandate of donors and NGOs has contributed towards reproducing a 'great divide' between traditionalists and western bushmen. It has been argued, however, that this divide is not simply imposed from above by NGOs and donors, but is also very much a product of local constructions of bushman identity and community.

San cultural revivalism is taking place within the context of a new politics of indigenous identity and cultural rights that is currently unfolding in South Africa. The stakes are being raised through tough competition over access to donor and state resources, including struggles for access to government salaries within a proposed Indigenous Council (*Inheemse Raad*), a KhoiSan equivalent of the existing House of Traditional Leaders. These recent developments have contributed towards exacerbating leadership struggles and social divisions amongst the Kalahari San. Such conflicts over traditional leadership and identity could also end up deflecting attention away from addressing the more mundane and material liveli-hood needs of these hyper-marginalised rural communities.

The ǂkhomani San land claim unfolded within this complicated post-apartheid political landscape. The gains made by ǂkhomani San and other indigenous groups in recent years would not have been possible during the apartheid era. There are a number of reasons for this, including the fact that San, Nama and Griqua were cat-egorised and interpolated as Coloured. The 'authentic San' were deemed 'extinct', and the Nama (Khoi) and Griqua were seen by the apartheid state to be part of an assimilated and hybrid Coloured population living in the Coloured Reserves of the Northern Cape (see Chapter 2). It is only in the post-apartheid period that people with San, Nama and Griqua ancestry have been able to publicly assert themselves as indigenous peoples with specific land, cultural and language rights. Despite refraining from entrenching indigenous rights in the constitution, the ANC gov-ernment has in fact addressed many of these claims through land restitution, by providing resources to promote Nama and San languages, and by addressing the question of traditional leadership. This political environment has enabled SASI and the San to make successful claims to land and cultural rights. While these claims have resulted in significant gains for this marginalised San community, a stress on primordial notions of San tradition and First People status has also had unintended consequences in terms of generating conflict between traditional and western bushmen, as well as running against the grain of donor and NGO ideas about the civic culture of liberal individualism, rights, duties and responsibilities. This chapter has attempted to examine the ambiguities and contradictions of these NGO and donor-driven double visions and local struggles over rights, citizenship, accountability, land, tradition, and identity.

Finally, the Human Rights Commission's (2004) documentation of intra-com-munity conflict, social fragmentation, desperation and chronic poverty at the new resettlement area in the Kalahari referred to at the beginning of this chapter, draws attention to the limited capacity of this post-apartheid indigenous peoples' move-ment to significantly transform ǂkhomani San lives and subjectivities. While the reinvention of San identity in the 1990s was highly effective in terms of enhancing the media visibility and political importance of this land claim, it did not create the conditions for effective livelihoods and forms of cultural and social capital neces-sary for poor people to make a decent living in the dry, red sands of the Kalahari. In many cases, ǂkhomani San beneficiaries of the land claim appeared to be just as poor and destitute as they were prior to the claim. Yet, as was mentioned ear-lier, Roger Chennels' effective use of cultural and intellectual property rights has created the possibility for accessing state, donor and big business resources and payments that can be used to revitalise and constitute community and livelihoods.

This ǂkhomani San case tells the story of the limited successes of attempts by SASI, a globally connected NGO, to establish an indigenous peoples' social movement in South Africa. This NGO–social movement partnership contributed towards promotion of both 'rights talk' and common conceptions of indigenous San identity that came into conflict in various ways. The next chapter draws attention tc a different type of NGO–social movement partnership, and highlights the ways in which local community networks and individual power brokers and gatekeepers belonging to the South African Homeless Peoples Federation (SAHPF) were able to circumvent and reinterpret some of the key democratic ideas and practices of the global social movement to which they belonged – the Slum Dwellers International (SDI). Chapter 4 draws attention to the successes and limits of the efforts of the SDI to promote practices of 'deep democracy' and 'grassroots globalisation' in the face of powerful local actors and networks in Phillipi township in Cape Town.

4

'Civil Society' & Popular Politics in the Postcolony
'Deep Democracy' & Deep Authoritarianism
at the Tip of Africa?

Introduction[1]

On 17 September 2002, about two hundred people from diverse race, class and ethnic backgrounds gathered at the Centre for the Book in Cape Town's city centre to hear the internationally known housing activist, Sheela Patel, talk about the work of an alliance of Mumbai-based slum dweller's federations that are part of the global network of the Slum Dwellers International (SDI). The audience included a large group of black South African women and young people from the South African Homeless People's Federation (SAHPF), activists, members of parliament, judges, academics and ordinary citizens. This was Patel's twentieth visit to Cape Town as part of a decade-long exchange programme between housing activists and slum dwellers from India, Thailand, South Africa and eleven other developing countries. Patel spoke of her organisation's strategies for empowering the urban poor in India – of the 'horizontal exchanges', savings schemes, 'toilet festivals',[2] self-enumeration and self-census exercises and various other 'empowerment rituals' deployed by these Indian women's federations. Patel concluded by noting

[1]   This chapter would not have been possible without the support and assistance of a number of people, especially Bettina von Lieres and Sarah Bologna. I would also like to thank Joel Bolnick, Ted Baumann, Leo Podlashuc, Diana Mitlin, Kathy Glover, Thami Maqulana, Thomas Koelble, David Chidester, and numerous members of the South African Homeless People's Federation such as Xolani and Buntu for their generous assistance. I would also like to thank Naison Ngoma, Ranjita Mohanty, Naila Kabeer, Alex Shankland, Lisa Thompson, John Williams, and John Gaventa and numerous other participants in the Development Resource Centre (DRC) project on Citizenship, Participation and Accountability. Thanks also go to the Human Sciences Research Council (HSRC) for supporting the research that went into this chapter.

[2]   For an excellent account of SDI's philosophy and practice see Leopold Podlashuc's doctoral thesis 'Class for itself? Shack/slum Dwellers International: the praxis of a transnational urban poor movement.' Faculty of Humanities and Social Sciences, University of Technology, Sydney, 2006. Also see Arjun Appadurai's (2002b) fascinating account of SAHPF's SDI partners in Bombay in which he analyses their rituals of 'toilet festivals' and 'the politics of shit'. He shows how a carnivalesque spirit of transgression and bawdiness prevails during toilet inspections in the presence of middle-class government and World Bank officials. This is interpreted by Appaduari as an attempt to redefine the private act of humiliation and suffering – shitting in the open – into a scene of technical innovation and self-dignification. It is seen as an innovative 'politics of recognition from below'.

that houses, savings, good governance and accountability were not the primary objectives of these slum dwellers' organisations. Instead, the aim was to create South–South poor people's networks in order to fight the isolation and disempowerment produced by conditions of poverty. SAHPF members, many of whom had visited India, spoke of their own experiences in establishing savings groups and building their houses in Cape Town's African townships. They spoke of how organising as a Federation – and as members of a social movement/NGO partnership – had assisted them in accessing the state housing subsidies. The Indian model of savings and housing federations had also provided these women with the leverage they needed to access state and donor resources. This town hall meeting in the heart of a still hyper-segregated post-apartheid city seemed to provide a glimpse into what Arjun Appadurai (2000; 2002b),[3] Judith Green (1999) and other SDI intellectuals refer to as grassroots globalisation and 'deep democracy'.

Three years after Patel's visit to Cape Town, the Cape Town SAHPF and its NGO partner, People's Dialogue (PD), were in a state of deep crisis as a result of financial mismanagement and serious conflict between middle-class professionals and the SAHPF's working-class leadership based at the Victoria Mxenge (VMx) Federation in Cape Town. Deep divisions also surfaced between the VMx leadership and rival federations in the Western Cape Province. As a result of these intractable conflicts, in 2005 it was decided to disband People's Dialogue. It had become apparent that the VMx leadership had accumulated extraordinary influence and power in ways that undermined the SDI's model for deep democracy, with its emphasis on non-hierarchical, decentralised leadership and grassroots mobilisation. Instead of promoting this SDI model, the VMx leadership had established a centralised style of leadership that tightly controlled federation resources in fundamentally anti-democratic ways. Whereas the SDI's model seemed to work well in India, and other parts of Asia and Africa, it had produced an authoritarian leadership in Cape Town's predominantly Xhosa-speaking township of Phillipi. Rather than viewing this state of affairs simply as a reflection of a political culture specific to the townships of the Western Cape, this chapter will argue that the VMx case study tells us something more general about the politics of patronage in the postcolony.

For NGO activists, academics, donors and policymakers, the emergence of social movements such as SDI reflects the burgeoning of a global civil society that offers prospects of a renewal and deepening of liberal democracy in the Global South. Yet, in many cases these well-intentioned civil society interventions end up looking like anything but 'deep democracy'. This chapter will show how attempts to deepen democracy through the SAHPF network ended up unwittingly reinforcing local power asymmetries and patronage networks. It demonstrates that the SDI model of deep democracy, when viewed from Cape Town's African townships, failed to produce 'horizontal networks' and democratic forms of social capital and

---

[3] I make reference to Appadurai's writings in this chapter because his ideas are extremely influential amongst intellectuals within the SDI network. His work is available on SDI websites and he regularly engages with key SDI leadership figures in India, South Africa and various other countries belonging to the SDI.

solidarity. Instead, it revealed the ambiguous, and at times highly contradictory, relationship between SDI's global vision of democracy and the everyday local realities and political practices of the community-based leadership of this social movement for the urban poor.

This chapter confines itself to a single federation, the Victoria Mxenge (VMx) scheme at Phillipi in Cape Town, and does not claim to generalise its findings to the hundreds of other federations spread throughout South Africa, India and many other parts of the Global South. It does, however, raise questions about the social experiments initiated by globally connected movements such as SAHPF. For instance, to what degree did the rank-and-file SAHPF members at VMx (Phillipi) share the official SDI ideology, and how did this ideology resonate with local political ideas and practices? Exploring these issues can throw light on the plethora of experiments in 'grassroots globalisation' and what is sometimes referred to as international civil society.

The World Bank, NGOs, donors, activists and anthropologists have become fascinated with global networks such as SDI. These social experiments are referred to in the literature as transnational advocacy networks (TANs), cross-border activism and examples of 'globalisation from below'.[4] These global networks are also increasingly recognised as playing a crucial role in the creation of an international civil society representing the needs of the poorer 80 per cent of the population of the world (now totalling 6 billion). For Arjun Appadurai (2002b), for example, through participation in these transnational networks 'the global and the local can become reciprocal instruments of the deepening of democracy' (ibid.: 25). These social movements, often in partnerships with NGOs, are seen to have found new ways of combining local activism with horizontal, global networking. But what happens when these models of horizontal networking land in settings characterised by vertical and centralised political cultures and styles of leadership?

The case study of the SAHPF-VMx draws attention to the Janus-faced character of 'civil society': its democratic and emancipatory face, as well as its illiberal and authoritarian underbelly. It also highlights the observation that for the popular classes in the Global South it is seldom possible to entirely avoid having to engage with the undemocratic and authoritarian political institutions and practices of uncivil society. Before turning to a discussion of the SAHPF, it is necessary to situate these experiments in 'deep democracy' and globalisation from below within the context of current debates on popular politics in the African postcolony.

---

[4]   Considerable scholarly and public policy attention has also been given to transnational advocacy networks (TANs) and globally connected social movements such as those affiliated to SDI. These developments are seen to have contributed towards a new form of politics or cross-border activism that enables citizens to work across national boundaries to advance their concerns to both national and transnational institutions (Beck 1995; Taylor 1996; cited in Jones and Gaventa 2002). The globalisation of the anti-globalisation movement has also become highly visible at mass demonstrations in numerous cities including Seattle, Davos, Genoa, Durban, Johannesburg, and Buenos Aires. Meanwhile, donors, academics and activists claim that there has been a paradigm shift from the well-worn mantra 'think globally, act locally' to the new rallying cry: 'think locally, *act globally*.' But it is not yet clear that the globally connected anti-globalisation demonstrations from Davos to Durban are indeed signs of the emergence of 'global civil society,' or that this constitutes what some refer to as a 'global associational revolution'.

Patronage politics in the Afromodern postcolony

Africa is persistently perceived as being plagued by patrimonialism, communitarianism and other political irrationalities. Analyses of the 'politics of the belly' and 'kleptocratic states' have become the staple of African studies (Bayart 1993; Bayart, Ellis and Hibou, 1999; Mbembe 2001). In sum, Africa has come to be seen as a place of undemocratic and illiberal politics and 'failed,' 'weak,' 'partial,' 'criminal' and 'shadow' states (see Migdal 1988; Reno 1995, cited in Roitman 2004: 193). As Celestine Monga puts it, Africa is 'the El Dorado of wild thought' (Monga 1996: 39, cited in Das and Poole 2004: 31).

Alongside this failed-state paradigm is a burgeoning scholarly literature that peddles images of the exotic 'Otherness' of Africa in which the continent is characterised by 'uncivil' societies awash in witchcraft, everyday violence, civil wars, corruption, disease, famine, and social, economic and political collapse and disintegration. While these phenomena do indeed exist in many parts of the continent, African states and political realities are far more complex and differentiated than these sweeping generalisations suggest. Neither are these political realities unique to the African continent.

While citizens in the West are portrayed as individualistic, increasingly cynical or depoliticised, Africans are represented as either primordial, 'tribal' subjects, or else as frenzied zombies driven to violence by occult forces and subjected to illiberal, irrational and tyrannical rulers. From this perspective, the prognosis for liberalism, democracy and rights in Africa looks very bleak indeed, notwithstanding the eagerness of Western donors to export this political system to the Third World.

The paradox of this donor-driven civilising mission is that, despite its desire to modernise and democratise the Third World, it reproduces images of its fundamental Otherness. This democracy industry, in its desire to promote Western-style democratic citizenship and governance, also tends to ignore how, in neo-liberal, post-colonial settings, the poor and marginalised are compelled to respond to uncertainty and radical contingencies on a daily basis. This requires multiple strategies that include clientelistic relationships as well as social mobilisation to claim rights from the state. In other words, everyday politics in the postcolony often comprises a complex mix of rights-based claims and strategic engagements with non-state actors and institutions, often of a non-democratic, violent and hierarchical nature. Donor-driven democratisation and governance programmes are unlikely to succeed unless they take cognisance of these hybrid political cultures.

Politics in Africa has been shaped by multiple political traditions, including colonial indirect rule, anti-colonial nationalism and varieties of liberalism, state authoritarianism and socialism. South Africa's ANC, for example, was established in 1912 as a liberal modernist nationalist organisation that challenged the contradictions between the purportedly universal principles of liberalism propagated by Europeans and the authoritarian and racist forms of colonial rule. After the Second World War, the ANC was increasingly influenced by both anti-colonial and socialist political traditions. By 1994, when democracy arrived, the ANC ruling party found itself subject to a post-Cold War, neo-liberal world order. While South Africa's version of liberal democracy differs in significant respects from contemporary Euro-American democracies, it also shares many features. It is only by investigating the specificities of the South African situation that it is possible to grasp the complex relationships between its 'local' specificities and its global or universal affinities.

Notwithstanding the thoroughly hybridised character of African modernities, political commentators and donors have persisted in reproducing a 'great divide' between Euro-American and African political realities. African communities continue to be perceived as being built upon the 'ethnic' foundations of primordialist political imaginaries and collectively shared myths of natural belonging. These communities also tend to be portrayed as characterised by involuntary membership and long-term, life-long commitments and solidarities. While African communities are understood to rely on narratives of cultural and historical continuity and coherence, the hyper-transient communities of the West appear to have no such requirements – anyone is free to sign up as long as you pay your membership fees! Maintaining these transitory experimental communities, however, requires considerable effort to avoid dissolution, whereas traditional communities appear to take on a naturalised sense of permanence.

This chapter challenges these age-old binaries by highlighting the difficulties SAHPF faced in creating and sustaining a social movement of the urban poor under South African conditions of chronic poverty, underdevelopment, racial and class inequalities, structural unemployment, disease, and violence. The SAHPF shows that South African society is not characterised by primordial ties of tradition and communal solidarity, but neither does it comprise atomised lone citizens of the variety that are deemed to inhabit modern Western democracies. Instead, South Africa is a modern state with a constitutional democracy that promotes liberal individualist notions of the rights-bearing citizens while also accommodating and protecting traditional leadership and African communitarian values. South Africa also has a strong modern economy and a large state bureaucracy that is capable of delivering services and resources to its citizens.[5] Activists from the PD and SAHPF were acutely aware of these realities, and this strongly influenced the forging of pragmatic strategies that sought to leverage access to these state resources. While scholars, donors and policy makers often struggle to grasp these hybrid postcolonial realities, activists are constantly challenged to develop new strategies to address these complexities. These strategies tend to be considerably more nuanced than the binary thinking of many of the donor think-tanks that drive the democracy industry (see Chapter 1).

---

[5] For example, since 1994 the ANC government has provided access to clean water for 9 million people, built 1.5 million houses, and installed electricity and telephone connections to more than 1 million homes. It has also constructed hundreds of new clinics that provide primary health care, desegregated medical services, made health services free to pregnant mothers and children under five years of age, and developed nutrition programmes that reach 5 million children. See Benatar, S. 2004. 'Health Policy Report: Health Care Reform and the Crisis of HIV and AIDS in South Africa'. *The New England Journal of Medicine* 351(1): 81–92; www.nejm.org

Seeing like the democracy industry: clientelism and other blindspots

One of the most glaring gaps in the academic and policy writing on democracy and 'civil society' is a serious engagement with popular forms of state and non-state clientelism and patronage that pervade everyday political life in many parts of the global South. There has instead been a tendency to valorise forms of citizenship and community participation that resonate with the normative preferences of researchers, NGOs, and donors, ignoring less normatively attractive vertical relations of exchange and political practice. It would seem, from this perspective, that to be a 'real citizen' it is necessary to refrain from being a client, as if clientelism were a deficit position, a form of negative or perverse social capital. In other words, only certain forms of agency are recognised within this highly normative democracy discourse. Yet, as this case study of SAHPF-VMx in Cape Town suggests (see below), clientelism is very much part of political life in many parts of the world today. Some of the NGOs and social movements discussed in this book have, however, recognised the need to strategically engage with these non-democratic and illiberal political discourses.

While clientelistic politics may indeed have negative and anti-democratic consequences, they remain dominant forms of political culture in many countries in the Global South. To deny clientelism's political salience on the basis of normative assumptions is clearly problematic for researchers, activists, NGOs, donors and governments alike. Such an approach obscures the complex ways in which citizens and clients straddle competing political logics, institutions and practices. The significance of claim-making as a client is particularly pervasive in developing countries where strategies of survival and well-being depend on the ability to establish multiple strategic relationships and become legible to a number of powerful actors, be they state functionaries, NGOs, religious and occult leaders and organisations, kinship groups, 'big men' or traditional leaders. While to outside observers these relationships may appear to reproduce dependency and disempowerment – the antithesis of liberal individualist conceptions of citizenship – they can also create the conditions for access to resources. These clientelistic relationships, whether they are with state functionaries, NGOs, donors, tribal elders, warlords, shacklords, or local power brokers, also allow citizen-subjects to make demands as clients of powerful patrons. Furthermore, should patrons fail to deliver, clients can exercise agency by shifting allegiance to another patron or acting to harm or undermine the legitimacy of the patron. Patrons need clients as much as clients need patrons, and this can produce a kind of mutual dependency, and a form of accountability within these relationships. In other words, patronage regimes do not necessarily obliterate individual agency.

These kinds of patronage regimes may indeed work for people in ways that a more abstract, distant citizen–state relationship cannot. In certain contexts they may also work more effectively than client–NGO relationships. This is especially evident in settings where the capacity of the state or NGO to deliver is severely constrained. By establishing clientelistic relationships with 'big men', including state functionaries and politicians, clients may be able to leverage access to state resources. It is therefore not surprising that, while the African National Congress (ANC) government promotes a liberal modernist constitutional democracy, in certain circumstances and contexts it operates in terms of patronage logics. However, this patrimonial state is also regularly subjected to accountability through the Constitutional Court, statutory bodies as well as the agency of its client-citizens. Local government restructuring in post-apartheid South Africa, for instance, is replete with examples of how members of poor communities are using patronage relationships, together with street action, and at times violent protest, to leverage access to housing, land and other state resources and services. For example, in 2006, during South Africa's local government elections, residents in Khutsong township, furious with the ANC government's decision over provincial demarcations, enforced a successful electoral boycott and burnt houses belonging to ANC candidates and party agents. Township activists claimed that the ANC government had not consulted the community over its decision to include Khutsong in North West Province, a historically impoverished part of the country. Rather than exercise their vote or engage in further deliberation, these traditionally ANC supporters took to the streets in what amounted to a successful, albeit violent and coercive, election boycott; only 300 out of 30,000 residents voted (*Mail & Guardian*, 3 March 2006).

These examples of citizen agency suggest that the relationship between 'the citizen' and 'the state' in many Third World settings seldom resembles the kinds of deliberative democratic models of citizen participation promoted by NGOs, donors and democracy think-tanks. In fact, it could be argued that people in poor neighbourhoods, whether in South Africa, India or Brazil, often stand to lose much by entering these deliberative spaces and abandoning patronage politics and popular demonstrations. Instead, it makes sense to engage simultaneously in multiple domains of politics, including those of the state, NGOs, religious organisations, and powerful patrons and 'big men'. The NGOs, activists and social movements discussed in this book have found themselves imbricated in these complex webs of relationships, solidarities, and networks, including those characterised by both democratic and clientelistic political logics and practices. Without a deep understanding of these political processes, it is likely that donor programmes will continue to be hijacked by political forces that may be more committed to profoundly authoritarian and illiberal styles of leadership.

How deep is 'deep democracy'?

Recent explosions of ethnic and religious-based conflicts throughout the world, including Africa, suggest that liberal individualist conceptions of citizenship are not the only game in town. Yet, in terms of conventional liberal democratic theory, citizenship is meant to erode local, 'ethnic' and communitarian hierarchies, statuses and privileges in favour of national jurisdictions and contractual relations based in principle on equality of rights and the individual rights-bearing citizen (Appadurai and Holston 1996). In other words, the liberal model of citizenship implies a self-interested and autonomous citizen-subject.[6] Anthropologists writing on post-

---

6   John Gaventa (2002: 4) points out that this construct has been 'critiqued by communitarians who argue

colonial African subjectivities (see Werbner 2002) have challenged this liberal individualist conception by arguing that the image of the 'lone citizen' fighting for his or her rights is generally at odds with African realities (see Chapter 1). Richard Werbner (2002) and Francis Nyamnjoh (2002), for instance, have noted that conviviality, intersubjectivity and interconnectedness are especially highly valued in contexts of vulnerability and uncertainty that characterise everyday life in many parts of Africa. These critiques of liberal individualism, which also appear in the documents of People's Dialogue and SDI, need to be taken particularly seriously in places like South Africa where, in certain settings, the liberal model of citizenship bears little relation to actually existing social and political realities.[7]

Critiques of liberal individualism come especially alive in post-apartheid South African debates on the role of traditional leaders in local government structures, customary law and land allocation (Comaroff and Comaroff 2005; Koelble and LiPuma 2005; Ntsebeza 2005; Robins 2005; Von Lieres 2005;). The ANC's modernist vision of a non-racial, non-sexist post-apartheid society underpinned by a liberal democratic Constitution, has been forcefully challenged by traditional leaders determined to hold onto political power and land ownership in the former ethnic homelands (Bantustans). This mode of traditional governance has its violent and authoritarian counterpart in South Africa's informal settlements and townships where warlord-politicians and powerful taxi owners, gangsters, and local businesspeople wield extraordinary political power and influence. It is here at the grassroots level that the visions of 'deep democracy' shared by Appadurai and SDI intellectuals are most likely to be contested. Viewing the SDI's project of grassroots globalisation from local spaces such as Cape Town's Phillipi township, highlights some of the most obvious challenges to social movement attempts to deepen democracy in South Africa and elsewhere in the South.[8]

---

[6] ...ntd that an individual's sense of identity is produced only *through* relations with others in the community of which she or he is a part' (ibid.). Gaventa notes that civic republican models of citizenship place more stress on people's political identities as *active citizens*, apart from their identities in localised communities (ibid.). This model emphasises individual obligations to participate in communal affairs through deliberative forms of democracy, in contrast to the liberal stress on representative democracy. As Gaventa notes, 'Recent work in contemporary citizenship theory attempts to find ways of uniting the liberal emphasis on individual rights, equality and due process of law, with the communitarian focus on belonging and the civic republican focus on processes of deliberation, collective action and responsibility. In so doing, it aims to bridge the gap between citizen and state by recasting citizenship as practices rather than given' (ibid.).

[7] While the activists belonging to People's Dialogue that I interviewed were indeed critical of liberal individualist models of citizenship, they were equally uncomfortable with communitarian forms of politics that violated individual rights and reinforced the centralisation of power through dominant networks and cliques (see the Victoria Mxenge case study). The challenge for them was how to mediate and reconcile these competing, and at times contradictory, political logics and cultures of politics.

[8] This liberal democratic project is also challenged by the retreat of citizens into race, class and ethnic laagers and communitarian solidarities. The difficulties the South African State has encountered in terms of providing jobs, health care (e.g., AIDS treatment) and social and economic security to the poor could also end up reinforcing and consolidating non-liberal, hierarchical and patriarchal traditional structures and client-patron relations. Such processes could contribute towards reproducing the contradictory logics of liberal and illiberal political cultures that currently characterise the South African political landscape (see Von Lieres, 2005).

Global citizens in local spaces: local is not always lekker![9]

These days concepts such as global citizenship, global civil society and globalisation from below are common currency and in constant circulation in academic, activist and donor and policy discourses (Appadurai 2001, 2002b). They have emerged in a neo-liberal global order in which the nation state is seen to be increasingly incapable of delivering resources in the form of enforceable rights to goods and services and political participation. In addition, the influence of multinational and intergovernmental institutions over people's lives calls for the acknowledgement of the need for accountability and rights to be enforceable across national borders (Beck 1995, cited in Jones and Gaventa 2002: 20). Even the World Bank has got in on the act with international conferences on 'connecting the local to the global'. Global connectivity has also been linked to calls from Third World leaders such as President Thabo Mbeki to 'narrow the digital divide'. Concepts such as 'digital citizenship' circulate notwithstanding the extremely limited distribution of cyber technology within developing countries.[10]

While terms such as 'global civil society' and 'global citizenship' and 'digital citizenship' conjure up optimistic images of Emanuel Castell's networked information societies, it would seem that for the vast majority of poor people in the developing world the benefits of global civil society seem elusive, and their social lives remain as parochial and isolated as ever. Whereas 'community' continues to suggest feelings of comfort, safety and security, it is often elusive, especially for the chronically poor who are in most need of its protection and security. For the poorest of the poor, the ghetto has become a space that represents 'the impossibility of community', a place of social disintegration, atomisation and anomie (Wacquant in Bauman 2001: 122); as a document on the SDI website puts it: 'poverty is a relentless isolator'. According to Wacquant, 'Whereas the ghetto in its classical form acted partly as a protective shield against the brutal racial exclusion, the hyper-ghetto has lost its positive role of collective buffer, making it a deadly machinery for naked social regulation and social isolation' (ibid.; see also Merry, 2001). Meanwhile the middle classes in the leafy suburbs retreat behind electrified fences, vicious dogs and private security companies and confine themselves to gated communities and mass private spaces such as megashopping malls and entertainment centres (Davis 1990; Robins 2003). Given these conditions of poverty, inequality and social segregation and isolation, what role can NGOs and social movements such as PD and SAHPF play in building

---

[9] *Lekker* is a widely used Afrikaans word for 'nice'. By using the phrase *local isn't always lekker*, I am referring to the quite obvious observation that terms like community can have a multiplicity of meanings. It can connote comfort, security and protection, but it can equally represent danger, threat and exclusion.

[10] Globally connected social movements have mushroomed that address a diverse array of issues including AIDS, medical technologies, biotechnology, the environment, indigenous land rights, Third World debt, trade liberalisation, housing, as well as struggles over abortion and gay rights and the cultural politics of racial, linguistic and ethnic pride. This rise in 'global citizen action' has been described in a vast and burgeoning academic literature as cross-border activism. However, relatively little reflection has gone into assessing exactly who belongs to this global citizenry and what these forms of belonging and global citizenship actually mean for diverse people in different parts of the world.

interconnectivities, networks, social capital and solidarities amongst the urban poor? What kinds of tensions and contradictions emerge out of their engagement with SDI's vision of 'deep democracy' and locally embedded forms of clientelism, conviviality, solidarity and intersubjectivity? In other words, what does SDI's version of grassroots globalisation look like from Cape Town's townships at the tip of Africa?

During the liberation struggle, activists sought to render the townships ungovernable as part of popular resistance to apartheid. These days post-apartheid city managers and government officials respond to demonstrations against evictions in the townships by calling for 'zero-tolerance' policing to re-establish governance in these 'unruly' communities. As a result, township residents who cannot afford to pay rent or electricity and water bills often have these services terminated or are evicted from their homes. Opposition to evictions, water and electricity cut-offs, or street demonstrations against poor state delivery of housing and services incur the wrath of the state. New social movements such as the Soweto Electricity Crisis Committee (SECC), Abahlali base Mjondolo (The Durban Shack Dwellers' Movement), the Anti-Eviction Campaign (AEC), the Anti-Privatisation Forum (APF), and the Concerned Citizen's Forum have mobilised township communities in popular struggles against evictions and cut-offs. These forms of community-based mobilisation have not always been appreciated by the ANC as courageous grassroots activism. Instead, they are often portrayed by government and ruling party officials as irresponsible behaviour instigated by 'the ultra-Left.' Meanwhile, black youth, once praised as courageous 'Young Lions' of the anti-apartheid struggle, are routinely represented in the media as the dangerous and ungovernable 'lost generation', prone to crime, drugs and violence. Working-class townships, once celebrated as spaces of heroic resistance to apartheid, are increasingly characterised by city officials and the media as places of social pathologies: crime, violence, illegal drug trade, gangsterism, disease, teenage pregnancies and substance abuse (see Robins 2002). These representations of township dystopias are produced under conditions of extreme racial and class inequalities that fuel middle-class fears that the urban poor will eventually rise up in revolt against their state of subjugation and abjection.

NGOs and social movements such as PD and SAHPF have daily encounters with forms of local power and authority that do not always follow democratic practices. These local community realities – the illiberal face of uncivil society – clash with SDI's vision of 'deep democracy' and global civil society. They also raise more general questions about the nature of civil society in the Global South. For instance, Partha Chatterjee (2004) argues that the middle classes are the bedrock of an Indian civil society that is constituted as an elite enclave that represents the popular classes, or what he calls 'political society'. In Chatterjee's (2004: 4) analysis, Indian 'civil society' refers to 'a closed association of modern elite groups, sequestered from the wider popular life of the communities, walled up within enclaves of civic freedom and rational law'. These elites constitute the relatively small educated, bourgeois section of the population in Third World countries. The majority of the world's population, Chatterjee argues, belong to the popular classes, and the state has to draw this class in through development and welfare projects of governmentality.

Chatterjee's understanding of Indian civil society, notwithstanding its binary logic and failure to acknowledge the porous and changing character of civil society, can perhaps explain the vast chasm between the SDI and PD conception of 'deep democracy' and the centralised and non-democratic political culture that emerged at the VMx Federation. It would seem that the NGO professionals from PD, as well as other co-authors of SDI's philosophy and practice, come from the relatively small elite enclave of the educated middle classes. By contrast, the SAHPF-VMx leadership that challenged PD came from working-class communities; being more embedded in popular politics and local political cultures, which includes clientelistic styles of popular leadership, meant they did not necessarily share the same political values as the middle-class NGO professionals who were generally responsible for elaborating SDI's sophisticated philosophy and practice.[11]

SDI keywords

Slum Dwellers International's philosophy and practice
A scan of SDI publications, including its website, provides a clear indication of the official ideological orientation and organisational practices of the SDI and its affiliates (see Podlashuc 2006).[12] The SDI literature reveals a deep scepticism of the role of experts and vanguards, and of the technocratic state's capacity to eradicate poverty and comply with its social contract to its citizenry. It is equally sceptical of the ability of traditional trade unions, left-wing political parties and rights-based social movements to provide the kind of long-term capacity-building that organisations of the poor require in order to strengthen themselves at the local level. The SDI is primarily concerned with building a social movement whose members have self-capacity, agency and autonomy. The anonymous author of the document cited below calls for poor communities to engage in practices of ***active citizenship*** rather than becoming passive recipients of development by experts, the state, or through party political patronage and largesse. Contrary to neo-liberal ideologues and free marketers, however, SDI ideology does not call for the dismantling or downsizing of the development state, but rather the empowerment of

---

[11] There are of course some striking exceptions. For instance, Jockin Apurtham, an Indian slum-dweller, has become a central leadership figure and organic intellectual within the SDI.

[12] See Leopold Podlashuc's 2006 doctoral thesis for a systematic discussion of the origins, influences and formation of SDI. Podlashuc's study of the SDI is an investigation of the philosophical underpinnings and organisational practices of this extraordinary transnational urban social movement. He argues that slum dwellers constitute a *lumpenproletariat* with the capability, through social movement activism, to acquire forms of critical consciousness and radical political subjectivity. His exploration of the ontology of SDI praxis includes an overview of the theoretical and philosophical strands that inform the SDI's praxis and modes of mobilisation. Podlashuc's theoretical exposition maps out the philosophical roots of SDI praxiology, through the writings of Antonio Gramsci, Karl Korsch, Georg Lukacs, the Frankfurt School of Critical Theory, Erich Fromm, Paulo Freire ('praxis of pedagogy'), Frantz Fanon and South African Black Consciousness theorist, Steve Biko. The study also focuses on the SDI's core operational rituals of Savings, Exchanges, and Federation, as well as its mobilising tools of Enumeration, House-modelling, House building and Sanitation, which are discussed later in the chapter.

poor communities to enable them to pressure and lobby the state to meet their own clearly-defined developmental needs.

> They [the SDI federations] see themselves as opponents of centralised state power, backed by these global agencies – the United Nations and the International Monetary Fund and the World Bank … They all share a common vision: that the State on its own cannot solve problems of poverty and underdevelopment. While the State, especially in Southern countries, has a monopoly on power, its very relationship to this power and to the local and global economy makes it a very weak instrument for the delivery of resources and services needed to eradicate poverty … [The SDI] constantly seeks situations that enable those who are affected by poverty to become organised and united in ever-expanding networks and to play a defining role in the way in which Governments and multilaterals discharge their obligations to the poor. This is in sharp contradiction to the rights-based social movements or the microfinance organisations, or even archaic social movements of the past, such as earlier rural and urban movements of the poor, including trade unions and left-wing political parties … SDI is an attempt to *move away from sporadic impulses to sustained, long-term investments in local federations* of the urban poor. SDI, as a network of these federations, opens opportunities at the international level in order to strengthen its member organisations. (SDI 2002: 1, emphasis added)

These SDI publications represent the federation affiliates and their members as belonging to a transnational citizenry of the urban poor, hence their use of the all too familiar slogan: 'think global, act local' (SDI 2002: 14). This 'cosmopolitan' perspective seeks solidarities and alliances of the urban poor across national, ethnic and religious lines. It appears to promote a sense of global citizenship rather than being confined to local, regional or national spaces and identities. SDI also represents the work of the federations as providing a clear alternative to mainstream development thinking and modern state development ideas and practices. Although SDI publications are critical of centralised, top-down state-driven development interventions, they do not follow the adversarial logic of anti-globalisation social movements. Instead, these statements seem to imply that through the combination of pressure, persuasion and negotiation, the state can be convinced, or if necessary shamed and pressured, into complying with its 'social contract' and developing 'poor-friendly' policies and urban development strategies.

The 'rituals' of the Federation savings schemes are meant to facilitate face-to-face encounters between members on a daily basis. It is these everyday interactions, along with the horizontal exchanges at the city, regional and international level, that are seen to create community networks and empower federations by strengthening the bargaining power in negotiations with officialdom, including the national, regional and local state. These rituals are performed to inscribe and embody the SDI's ideology of 'building people not things'. Savings schemes are meant to build both social capital and houses. SDI's approach to social capital, which differs quite significantly from conventional political science definitions (Putnam 1993), hinges on the fact that about 90 per cent of members are women. This gendered composition of the federations is perceived to be an advantage for social mobilisation since women are generally the de facto managers of poor households, with the household being the primary site of social reproduction. The following section shows how People's Dialogue has elaborated its theories of intervention based on these conceptions of social capital. It lays the groundwork for later discussions on the dangers of reifying 'positive' and 'progressive' social capital in local spaces characterised by undemocratic and authoritarian politics.

'Deep democracy' is a keyword in SDI organisational discourse. Arjun Appadurai's (2002b) work on SDI-affiliated housing activist groups in Mumbai draws attention to the emancipatory possibilities that globalisation presents in terms of deepening democracy and facilitating and strengthening cross-border activism and transnational advocacy networks. According to Appadurai (ibid.) these transnational SDI networks provide the possibility of deepening democracy through 'new horizontal modes for articulating the deep democratic politics of the locality'. Borrowing from an eclectic mix of John Dewey's pragmatist philosophy, Appadurai's writings, organisational development and whole systems theories, the PD and SDI's conceptualisation of 'deep democracy' highlights the organising principle and image of the network and 'the interconnected web of social actors'. This theorisation of 'deep democracy' borrows freely from diverse literatures including social capital, interpersonal communication, conflict resolution, learning organisations, communitarian and community participation theories. 'Deep democracy' is presented as an alternative to the liberal individualist conception of the citizen as 'an autonomous agent seeking to defend and expand his or her own piece of the pie [i.e., rights and interests] against other autonomous interests mediated by government structures to reduce conflict' (People's Dialogue 2003: 19). This challenges both the liberal democratic idea of the citizen as an autonomous rights-bearing subject, as well as essentialist and reified understandings of community and culture. This conception of 'deep democracy' is outlined in an unpublished PD document (ibid.).

> In deep democracy, citizenship is conferred by personal engagement – not just by revealing individual preferences through voting and rational choice, but by exercising the democratic arts of participation. It is based on public conversation, where one begins to listen to and know the 'other'. It becomes the enfranchisement of the self in daily life, transforming one's self identity into one of inclusion in, and responsibility for, an expanding circle of community. In contrast, we wish to posit the idea of deep democracy, in order to emphasise the social nature of the human – the idea that a person's identity is derived from his or her relationships with others. The image of the autonomous self-interested individual gives way in this alternative view to the image of the network, the interconnected web of existence that defines individuals in relationship to each other and defines institutions as an expression of the nature of the connections in the web. Deep democracy, as we see it, does not privilege the concept of community by reifying it into a single set of values. (People's Dialogue 2003: 19)

So how has the SAHPF embarked upon building 'deep democracy' in South Africa? With the steady support of its NGO partner, SAHPF, also known in Xhosa as *uMfelandawonye waBantu BaseMjondolo*, has grown into a 100,000 strong post-apartheid community-based organisation (CBO) – perhaps even a social movement in the making – that is both locally embedded and globally connected. The SAHPF-PD and SDI website documents reveal that these organisations are concerned with building local–global solidarities and forms of social capital that challenge 'expert' forms of knowledge and power. This website literature also draws attention to debates on various strategies for negotiating and lobbying with official-dom to access state resources and shift the balance of power between poor people and hierarchical, technocratic and bureaucratic states. What this all suggests is that globalisation is not only a source of structural disempowerment for millions of poor people in developing countries, but it also offers opportunities for creative financial, technical, cultural and social transactions and interactions between pro-fessionals, activists, state officials, donors and hundreds of thousands of homeless people and shack dwellers from Cape Town to Calcutta and beyond. But what kind of 'deep democracy' is emerging through these global exchanges?

Case study of Victoria Mxenge (VMx) Federation, Phillipi, Cape Town

The SAHPF-PD partnership was formed in 1991 and comprises mostly black Afri-can members, of whom more than 85 000 (85%) are women. It is part of the SDI network of affiliates ranging in size from a few hundred in Zambia to more than a million-and-a-half in India (SDI 2002: 1). The stated objective of the SDI federa-tions is for members to assume 'ownership of problems and the identification of local solutions that are participatory and inclusive [and] by doing so they auto-matically create new nodal points of governance, in which organised communities of the urban poor assume their rightful place as development actors' (SDI 2002: 14). The SAHPF slogan: 'We do not collect money, we collect people,' captures the organisation's concern with social capital. Drawing largely upon the Indian experience over the past two decades, the SAHPF-PD partnership promotes daily savings as a ritual that produces high levels of participation and mutual interac-tion between federation members – these daily encounters are perceived to be the social glue that binds communities. In addition, through investing limited funds, members have a material stake in their organisation and its decision-making. Not only do daily savings encourage regular interaction but they also create a space for the central participation of women in informal settlements and townships that tend to be dominated by patriarchal local structures. It is also meant to shift the balance of power and expert knowledge from technocratic and hierarchical state structures to local, decentralised federations. Savings and loans also enable fed-erations to develop capacity to manage and control finance and to display this local competence to the outside world. Members learn housing design, construction and finance, layout design, brick making, toilet construction, crafts and a range of other competencies including bookkeeping, census enumeration and information gathering (for example, self-surveys), methods for identifying vacant land through physical mapping and visits to the deeds offices, and the development of negotia-tion skills in order to secure land from the state. These activities are consciously framed as public performances of local competence and innovation. This has a number of purposes including posing a challenge to existing class cultures and beliefs about where expertise lies. It is an expression of *a politics of visibility and a public demonstration of 'autogovernmentality' or 'governance from below'* (see Appadurai 2002b, my emphasis).

Horizontal exchange is perhaps one of the most important of these rituals because of its ability to foster direct learning experiences from peers as opposed to the usual expert-driven methods of formal training. These visits also facilitate the creation of new transnational solidarities and networks, as well as being a catalyst for cross-cultural reflection and analysis by federation members. However, this chapter draws attention to the gap between the official ideology and 'praxiology' of the SDI and PD on the one side, and the everyday practices and local political cultures of one of the SAHPF affiliates, the Victoria Mxenge (VMx) Federation in Phillipi, Cape Town.

VMx is a low-income housing scheme situated on the outskirts of Cape Town. As a women's organisation that has been able to build significant numbers of houses, together with donor, NGO and state support, it has captured the imagination of tourists, government officials, NGOs, academics, diplomats, politicians and international figures such as Hillary and Bill Clinton. VMx Housing Project comprises single and double-story brick houses with neat gardens. It can be described as a post-apartheid low-income housing showpiece. These VMx houses are noticeably larger than the million tiny government subsidy houses built in South Africa's black townships since 1994. What is particularly interesting about this project is that for more than a decade its members have travelled to various parts of Africa, Asia and Latin America to meet with housing and savings organisations They are members of the SDI network of slum dweller organisations based in 14 countries and including such cities as Bombay, Calcutta, Nairobi, Bangkok, Karachi and Bogota. This global network seems to embody what is increasingly seen to be the emergence of an international civil society of global citizens.

VMx comprises predominantly working-class black African women who belong to savings schemes that are affiliated to the SAHPF, a national organisation that works in partnership with the PD, a Cape Town-based NGO comprising urban planning professionals. SAHPF is a women's organisation of the urban poor that is involved in a wide range of activities including savings clubs, housing and land issues, income-generation projects, community policing, AIDS intervention and so on.

People's Dialogue: Beyond rights talk?

> We are doing the daily savings not only to collect money but to collect the lives of the people. We do this so that they can know what is happening next door, what is happening today and tomorrow, how I can help, how we can involve each other daily. (Member of SAHPF, Phillipi, Cape Town, July 2002)

> The language of the Federation is saturated with [social capital] imagery: 'We build houses in order to build people'; 'we don't collect money, we collect people'. That is all over the show. (Joel Bolnick, Director and founder of People's Dialogue, the NGO partner of SAHPF, Observatory, Cape Town, July 2002)

PD and SAHPF define their objectives and ideological commitments in similar terms to other SDI affiliates. While the SAHPF shares these objectives and methodologies, there are certain localised dimensions to SAHPF savings schemes and leadership styles. Before discussing these localised practices, it is worthwhile drawing attention to the ideological orientation of PD, the NGO supporting the SAHPF.

The PD manifesto presented at the launch of the SAHPF on 21 March 1994 presents a 'radical' critique of the state and technocratic development. The highly polemical and poetic language of this PD document represents a strident critique of what is perceived to be the inevitable rise of the post-apartheid technocratic state. Barely a month after the tumultuous celebrations of the ANC's landslide victory in the first democratic elections of April 1994, the PD message is one of profound scepticism and distrust of the intentions of the new political and bureaucratic elite. The anonymous author warns that 'now that the Great Cause has been won, the average men and women in this land will witness the gross spectacle of politicians and other elites [using] the Cause to further their own personal hunger for power ... The State will use an army of technocrats and planners, equipped with the Great Cause, to control the social life of its subjects ... Their primary concern will be the circulation of things, and of human beings trapped in a world of things: cars, trains, commodities, sewerage. Poor people have to try to tear these topological chains asunder.' This anti-development language is suggestive of a radical alternative to 'development as usual'. Whereas these days PD works in close partnership with the ANC government, the PD's early manifestos represent a radical critique of state-led technocratic development reminiscent of recent post-development critiques (Escobar 1995; Sachs 1992).

Although current PD discourse can be characterised as critical engagement with government and 'development', PD nonetheless remains critical of state- and private sector-driven low-income housing delivery that fails to build poor people's capacity. Beneficiaries of state subsidy housing are provided with a physical structure but not the means to survive under conditions of extreme poverty. As PD respondents noted, in many cases unemployed recipients of the government housing subsidies end up renting or selling their subsidy houses for extremely low prices and moving back into informal settlements because the houses are too small and they cannot afford to extend using formal building materials, and/or they cannot afford to pay rates and service fees.[13] These product-driven housing delivery schemes also tend to reproduce relations of dependency and passivity amongst development beneficiaries ('the poor'): houses become 'projects' and 'products' rather than opportunities for long-term income generation and community building. The PD response has been to concentrate on direct, experiential learning and capacity-building rather than a narrow focus on housing delivery. Although securing finance, land and housing remains central to PD's approach, there has been a growing recognition of the need to return to SDI first principles, that is to build social capital by addressing a range of other issues including health, income generation, education, and youth development.

A PD proposal to begin a process of collecting statistics on HIV/AIDS prevalence within the federations revealed the influence of SDI theorising on the knowledge–power nexus, especially the role of censuses, statistics and surveys

---

[13] In 2008 a government housing subsidy consisted of R43,000 for the top structure only. In addition, beneficiaries received land and a serviced site at no cost to them.

in the reproduction of bureaucratic state power. Instead of resisting these forms of state power, the SDI affiliated federations sought to appropriate and recast these bureaucratic practices and use them as leverage for accessing state resources, for instance health care resources and AIDS treatment.[14] Self-enumeration and information gathering are also seen as crucial for engaging the State on more equal terms and holding it accountable to its citizens. These practices reflect a sophisticated understanding of the political and bureaucratic machinations of the modern State. By appropriating these rituals of bureaucratic State power, the federations acquire leverage in their negotiations with the State to secure resources such as housing and health.

In an anonymous PD document circulated to the South African federations, the author/s draw attention to the potentially emancipatory logics of practices of enumeration, censuses and surveys traditionally associated with the state. What emerges is a sophisticated re-reading of Foucault. The document entitled, 'Some notes on enumeration', questions certain Foucaultian critiques of governmentality that suggest that these state technologies inevitably buttress bureaucratic state power (Escobar, 1995), and are part of the repressive surveillance apparatus of the modern state (Scott, 1998). Whereas James Scott (ibid.) and Arturo Escobar (ibid.) portray these practices as bureaucratic forms of state domination and disciplinary power that render populations legible and susceptible to state processes of governmentality, the SAHPF-PD 'rituals' of self-enumeration are precisely about rendering the federation members *more legible to the state* in order to lobby for access to state resources. People's Dialogue intellectuals and their SDI partners suggest that there is nothing inherent in such state practices that pre-determine the outcomes of their application. However, while these SDI intellectuals have fashioned sophisticated tools such as self-enumeration for empowering SAHPF members, there appears to be a widening gap between SDI's official ideology and the ideas, desires, practices and commitments of the federation leadership and ordinary members.

Mind the gap: global ideologies and local realities

During interviews with PD and SAHPF-VMx members it became clear that there was a vast chasm between SDI official ideology and the ideas and practices of VMx leaders and members from Phillipi, Cape Town. While PD endorsed SDI thinking that stressed the importance of horizontal relations of trust and non-hierarchal and decentralised political structures and practices within and between federations, by 2002 the SAHPF national leadership in Cape Town had established highly centralised decision-making structures. This leadership was unwilling to relin-

---

[14] PD's thinking on how to approach the AIDS pandemic is a mirror onto the SDI's theory and practice. Rather than attempting to address HIV/AIDS treatment through litigation or by recruiting medical specialists and experts, PD sees its task as that of mobilising Federation communities so that they can leverage the state to comply with its social contract with its citizens and provide treatment to federation members. This is to be done by collecting AIDS-related data from federation members. By drawing on rituals of 'self-enumeration' and the power of statistics and the survey, the federation hopes to obtain strategic data that is currently not at the disposal of the state. This data can then be used by the federation to pressure the government to come up with concrete programmes to treat its members. This is very different to the litigation strategies and rights-based approaches of the Treatment Action Campaign (TAC) discussed in Chapter 5.

quish its control and authority over 'junior' federations, resulting power cliques and patronage networks that allowed certain individuals to act as gatekeepers. A member of PD suggested that the VMx Federation leadership was as hierarchical, centralised, violent and intolerant of competition as the neo-traditional male leadership structures that emerged in many urban and rural informal settlements throughout South Africa. He made the comparison between the current federation leadership and the neo-traditional and patriarchal leadership structures that emerged in Crossroads during the 1980s (see Cole 1987; Robins 1998). In addition to allegations of undemocratic practices and centralised political leadership, some SAHPF members accused the leadership of financial mismanagement. This culminated in general disillusionment with savings schemes and large-scale withdrawal of federation members from participation in these schemes. As PD's Cathy Glover put it, 'The federation has still been very successful in securing land in the city and initiating housing developments' but once people get these resources they often see no reason for continuing to belong to savings schemes and they tend to withdraw from federation activities.

The national leadership style of the SAHPF, which was based at VMx (Phillipi) in the Western Cape, contradicted the liberal democratic and egalitarian visions of SDI and People's Dialogue. However, it proved to be extremely difficult to alter these hierarchical political styles and power dynamics. This was especially the case at the showpiece Victoria Mxenge Federation, which was regularly visited by dignitaries, donors and government officials. One strategy advocated by PD in order to decentre and dismantle these concentrations of power was to regularly reinvent the organisational structure of the federations, for example by means of rotational leadership and by resuscitating local savings schemes and devolving decision-making powers to these schemes. According to Bolnick, it is necessary to constantly reinvent and restructure the organisation to prevent the ossification and consolidation of local power nodes and community structures. As Bolnick explained in an interview: 'On the one level, since 1994 when the Federation was formed, we have triggered a process where the Federation structures have changed four times: at national, regional and local [levels]. It has not been an easy role at all … Every time contradictions emerge inside the Federation, our response has been not to change the leadership, but to change the structure and in that way to change the leadership … So that is how the reinvention process happens.' These initiatives, however, encountered fierce opposition from a powerful SAHPF-VMx leadership that was determined to hold onto power and to resist attempts to decentralise the decision-making structures. This contributed towards ongoing clashes between PD and the SAHPF-VMx leadership, culminating in the closing down of PD in 2006 and the breakaway from the SAHPF to form a new organisation, the Federation of the Urban Poor (FEDUP). Moreover, it seemed that the global exchanges merely served to reinforce the social power and prestige of the leadership at the expense of the rank-and-file members.[15] It also contributed towards undermining the objectives of the SDI philosophy. Ted Bauman, the Executive Director of PD's Utshani

---

[15] Youth also complained that the VMx leadership, comprising a group of veteran ANC Women's League members, sidelined them and undermined any initiatives that VMx youth attempted to establish.

Fund reflected on these problems at Cape Town's VMx Federation:

> In Cape Town ... the local SAHPF leadership, based at the well-known Victoria Mxenge development, constructed an elaborate structure of control over resources, decision-making, and access to housing opportunities for ordinary SAHPF members all over the city. There is always an incentive for community leaders to position themselves as 'gatekeepers', controlling access to outside resources. One reason the SAHPF was founded was to combat this phenomenon by mobilising ordinary women savers to exercise their own decision-making rather than rely on 'leaders' to act as champions on their behalf. Over the years it became clear that some Cape Town SAHPF leaders, who appeared to embrace this vision rhetorically, in practice sought gatekeeping power for themselves. They no longer sought to mobilise ordinary women into savings groups, or help them to identify and act on their development options. Instead, they positioned themselves as 'champions' of a passive mass of the poor, fighting on their behalf to extract resources from the NGO. In return for this 'delivery', these 'champions' could extract rewards: power and material benefits for themselves. Sometimes this fight could be very dirty. By being too free with subsidy prefinance loans and other NGO resources, therefore, we had unconsciously reinforced the very conditions we sought to overcome. And as long as Utshani Fund continued to work through these leaders, we reinforced their position and thereby undermined our own development vision and mission. This was the antithesis of our vision and mission. (Bauman 2006)

There were numerous other divergences between the desires, agendas and objectives of the NGO and its CBO partner. For instance, the PD, like the SDI and its Indian affiliates, believed that long-term processes of creating and scaling-up of social capital and community building was more important than either rights-based approaches or product-driven concerns such as housing construction. However, this developmental vision was not always shared by SAHPF members, many of whom disappeared once they received the object of their desire – the subsidy house. Consequently, unlike their counterparts in India, many South African federation members did not buy into daily savings and other federation rituals and modes of building social capital.

One of the possible reasons for this difference between South African and Indian federations is that the latter seem to recruit the poorest of the poor whereas the SAHPF's working-class members are generally relatively well-off, when compared to their Indian counterparts. Many of these SAHPF members envisage participation in SAHPF as a way of networking with NGOs and state officials in order to access state and donor resources such as a formal brick house. They also sought technical knowledge and professional and leadership skills that would equip them in their quest for upward socio-economic mobility. Unlike the post-colonial situation of their Indian counterparts, social transformation programmes and affirmative action policies in post-apartheid South Africa have indeed created opportunities for skilled black women in the business, NGO and the public sectors. Membership of organisations such as PD and SAHPF became a conduit towards such resources and upward social mobility. The motivations for belonging to a federation in Bombay and Cape Town were clearly very different. This explains why savings rituals and other SDI practices that work well amongst the urban poor and structurally unemployed in Bombay failed to take off in Cape Town, a relatively wealthy city with a small population.

Another key area of difference relates to the political culture of the South African Federations. While these organisations were meant to be non-party political, a number of the leadership figures were seasoned ANC Women's League veterans who were deeply enmeshed in local, regional and national ANC networks. Further, whereas PD believed in critical engagement with the government, many of the ANC-aligned SAHPF leadership were less inclined to criticise the ANC government and leadership. Instead, a number of SAHPF leaders were prepared to allow federation networks to be used as ANC political resources. In addition, unlike their Indian partners, South African federation members tended to view the ANC government as a powerful patronage machine that could be accessed through party political contacts and channels. This perception of a powerful state was reinforced by the reality of the R16,500 state housing subsidies. The state was not only perceived to be a powerful provider of material resources, but also a repository of technical expertise and know-how. This SAHPF perception of the power of the technocratic state was very different to the anti-technicist, anti-hierarchical, anti-project and anti-bureaucratic perspective of PD and SDI. Whereas PD and SDI produced eloquent anti-technocratic tracts that challenged the expert/client relationship, it seemed that rank-and-file federation members, as well as the leadership, were not always as committed to this anti-technocratic post-development agenda.

PD practitioners and SAHPF members openly acknowledged the gap between SDI's 'global ideology' and the everyday realities that federation members experienced, and that not all federation members embraced the SDI development paradigm. This was particularly evident when federation members withdrew from regular participation in savings schemes upon the completion of the construction of their houses. These competing understandings of development permeated many aspects of PD's involvement with the SAHPF. For example, the PD and SDI website and newsletters advocated long-term capacity building, whereas the SAHPF members and leadership tended to stress housing delivery. This focus on housing infrastructure was often at the expense of less tangible outcomes such as social capital, democratic and accountable governance, and social fabric developments such as recreational spaces and crèches.

Despite these deviations from the SDI's objectives and methodologies, the VMx Federation had successes in attracting international media attention, donors and visiting dignitaries such as Hillary Clinton. This gap between SDI/PD official ideology and the everyday practices of SAHPF members may lie in the very different historical experiences of the South Africans and their Indian counterparts. Whereas the Indian organisations, for instance the National Slum Dwellers Federation (NSDF), have been around since the mid-1970s, the SAHPF–PD partnership was only established in the early 1990s. In addition, while the Indians have had five decades to come to terms with the limits of liberation and state-driven development, the South African federations are relative newcomers to democracy, and have far more faith in the capacity of the modern development state to address poverty. This faith is not entirely misplaced as the South African state does indeed have the capacity to hand out large development resources, for example the housing subsidies. As a result, many of the SAHPF members bought into government patronage politics and technocratic state development visions rather than striving towards becoming more self-sufficient through long-term investment in building social and financial capital (through daily savings, for example). These 'expectations of modernity' (Ferguson, 1999) could perhaps also explain why local patronage and centralised leadership practices emerged at VMx.

Conclusion

Although the VMx Federation, with the assistance of NGO professionals in PD, managed successfully to access state housing subsidies, it failed to produce the kinds of horizontal networks and forms of social capital and democratic practice envisaged by the SDI and PD leadership. Whereas not all federation members saw themselves as belonging to a rights-based social movement, the SAHPF drew on mass mobilisation to leverage government into converting its rhetoric on 'the right to housing' into reality. However, when it came to the SDI's vision about 'deep democracy,' there was a glaring gap between SDI rhetoric and SAHPF realities. In addition, whereas the SDI sought to create forms of 'social capital' through savings, in many cases federation members 'jumped ship' once they got their houses. Contrary to the democratic ethos of SDI, federation leaders at VMx became power brokers and gatekeepers in order to accumulate personal resources and power.

The chapter has argued that these developments can be explained by taking into account the specific political and economic context within which social movements such as the South African federations operate. Whereas in India federations appear to have a good record when it comes to mutual cooperation and savings, South African federations such as VMx are notorious for the high levels of misappropriation of funds, distrust and intense conflict. These differences have a lot to do with the high stakes involved in the South African development game, as well as a particularly rapacious and individualistic made-in-SA brand of neoliberal capitalism. Many SAHPF leaders and rank-and-file members recognised that joining VMx could be a ticket to a state housing subsidy as well as financial loans. Since Indian federations do not have access to such sizeable resources there is more of an imperative to develop the kinds of social capital – wealth in people – that SDI and PD advocate. By contrast, South Africa is a country of housing subsidies, where black economic empowerment (BEE) millionaires seem to emerge overnight and where extraordinary wealth is visible everywhere. Desire to access these state resources and sources of instant wealth appear to undermine attempts by social movements to build long-term social capital. It is within this context that housing activists have sought to embed the SDI philosophy of social capital formation.

This chapter also investigated what SDI's official ideology and everyday practices (rituals such as 'daily savings', 'horizontal exchange' and 'self-enumeration') actually meant to rank-and-file SAHPF members from Cape Town's Victoria Mxenge Housing Scheme. This study suggests that the forms of social capital and horizontal networks developed through these SDI and PD rituals contributed towards solidarities and collective action at local, regional, national and global levels. However, despite SDI and PD's commitments towards deepening democracy, not all VMx Federation members in Cape Town shared this long-term vision of building 'deep democracy'. For some federation members the attainment of 'the product' (land or the house) led to decisions to bail out of 'community'. In addition, the Victoria Mxenge case study showed that some SAHPF leadership figures used their global connections, ANC networks and forms of social capital to strengthen their positions as gatekeepers and powerbrokers. PD workers had to try to reconcile these gaps and contradictions between the SDI's official ideology and the everyday realities and cultures of politics at Phillipi and other townships in South Africa.

These findings question an uncritical celebration of the SDI's brand of grass-roots globalisation. Instead, it would appear that the SDI's experiments in 'deep democracy' have to be situated within specific localities, historical moments and political trajectories. For instance, the Indian and South African experiences look very different. 'Deep democracy', whether in Africa or Asia, remains an unfinished and ongoing project characterised by setbacks and defeats as well as victories and progress. The successes of the SAHPF in establishing communities such as Victoria Mxenge, for example, suggest that some of these housing federations are indeed capable of addressing the shortcomings and deficits of the (neo)liberal state and liberal individualist conceptions of the citizen as an autonomous agent. At the same time, the adoption and reconfiguration of these SDI democratic innovations in Phillipi produced undemocratic outcomes that required constant NGO inter-vention, including the reinvention of leadership structures as a means of rotating leadership. There was, however, constant tension between the local impetus to consolidate the VMx leadership, and calls from individuals within PD to rotate the leadership. These conflicts culminated in the PD's director eventually moving to another programme in the SAHPF, and a key VMx leader being co-opted into PD. This did not resolve the problems and PD was eventually shut down.

It may well be that the urban and rural poor in South Africa, living as they do under the harsh, uncertain and vulnerable conditions of neo-liberal capital-ism, are obliged to try out all sorts of alternatives including liberal rights that stress individualism and communitarian commitments that valorise intersubjectiv-ity and interconnectedness (Werbner 2002). Survival under such conditions may also require forms of collective belonging and solidarity that at times appear to be undemocratic and contradict liberal individualist conceptions of citizenship, rights, duties and responsibilities.

Sanitised and romantic versions of 'deep democracy', 'global citizenship' and the 'virtuous poor' are likely to obscure these contradictions and gaps between rhetoric and realities. They are also likely to ignore the shadow side of social exper-iments in 'grassroots globalisation' whether in India or South Africa. Some of the writings of Appadurai, for example, create the impression that SDI rituals such as daily savings and horizontal exchange embody deeply felt commitments to col-lective survival and solidarity amongst the millions of urban poor in Indian cities such as Mumbai (Bombay). Although the Indian side of the SDI story is no doubt considerably more complex and uneven, it does seem to provide a stark contrast to the hierarchical, centralised and authoritarian political cultures of Phillipi, Cape

Town. Notwithstanding the democratic deficits documented in the VMx case, PD and SAHPF were nonetheless highly successful in mobilising rights to state resources by leveraging access to housing subsidies and securing donor funding that financed the building of thousands of houses in Phillipi, and elsewhere in South Africa. Mobilising rights and social and economic resources under conditions of extreme poverty and marginalisation can indeed turn out to generate the kinds of tensions and contradictions that emerged at the Victoria Mxenge Federation.

5

AIDS, Science & the Making of a Social Movement
AIDS Activism & Biomedical Citizenship in South Africa

Introduction[1]

> It was not AIDS that was killing our loved ones, the dominant analysis went. It was witchcraft. Fingers were pointed at suspected neighbours.
>
> (Thokozani Mtshali, *Sunday Times*, 28 April 2002)

> The biggest challenge for doctors in rural KZN is getting HIV-positive women to ask for treatment: A bitter pill to swallow.
>
> (*Mail & Guardian*, 23 August 2002)

> This monograph discusses the vexed question of HIV/AIDS ... It also accepts that the HIV/AIDS thesis [is] informed by deeply entrenched and centuries-old white racist beliefs and concepts about Africans and black people ... In our own country, the unstated assumption about everything to do with HIV/AIDS is that, as a so-called 'pandemic', HIV/AIDS is exclusively a problem manifested among the African people.
>
> (*Castro Hlongwane*, March 2002)

> African children's faces have been paraded in the media in the name of giving a face to AIDS. I agree the disease must be given a face – but it should be human, not African ... Parading African children in the media adds to the stigma already suffered by those infected and affected by HIV/AIDS.
>
> (Phumzili Simelela, *Mail & Guardian*, 6 December 2002)

This chapter focuses on how South African AIDS activists and government interpreted and responded to the AIDS pandemic. In South Africa responses to HIV/AIDS have included forms of activism that, like the transnational housing activism case study in Chapter 4, could best be described as 'globalisation from below'

[1] This chapter benefited from the generous comments and contributions of a number of people especially Sarah Bologna, Nathan Geffen, Ian Scoones, Melissa Leach, Tobias Hecht, Kees van der Waal, Lyla Metha, Chris Colvin, and Zackie Achmat and countless TAC activists who have been the inspiration for this research project. I would also like to thank John Gaventa and numerous other participants in the joint School of Government, University of the Western Cape and Institute for Development Studies, Sussex University project on Citizenship, Participation and Accountability. I would also like to thank Jonathan Shapiro for allowing us to use his fantastically insightful HIV/AIDS cartoons. Finally, I would like to thank Lauren Muller for consistent support and encouragement.

(Appadurai 2001). The Treatment Action Campaign (TAC), the major AIDS activist organisation in South Africa, was founded by Zackie Achmat in 1998, and in 2001 TAC and *Médecins sans Frontières* (MSF – Doctors Without Borders) established South Africa's first and largest anti-retroviral (ARV) treatment programme at Khayelitsha, Cape Town. At the time the South African Government was resolutely against providing ARVs in the national public health system. TAC and MSF drew on rights to health care and mainstream AIDS science in a prolonged battle for access to cheap generic drugs. In response, President Mbeki and AIDS dissident supporters drew on arguments about 'Big Pharma' conspiracy theories in which TAC was portrayed as a front for profiteering pharmaceutical companies that were using Africans as guinea pigs to experiment with their toxic and lethal medicines. Underlying President Mbeki's position was a belief that AIDS activists and scientists were complicit in a racist assault on the dignity of Africans, an onslaught that portrayed African (male) sexualities as dysfunctional and dangerous. The media responded by portraying TAC and President Mbeki as occupying diametrically opposed positions in a raging battle between scientific truth and irrationality.

In their struggles for AIDS treatment, TAC and MSF responded to the pandemic in ways that drew on mainstream AIDS science and biomedicine, but they also went well beyond conventional biomedical approaches. These extra-medical activities included grassroots mobilisation in South Africa's townships, litigation against the global pharmaceutical industry and the South African Government, and the establishment of treatment support groups and campaigns that involved translating and mediating biomedical and rights discourse. In the course of these diverse activities TAC and MSF's approach confronted 'dissident' and 'denialist' views that persistently questioned mainstream AIDS science and treatment technologies.

This case study shows how AIDS activists, together with a global community of scientists, health professionals and journalists, drew on arguments about rights and responsibilities and moral and scientific truth in their responses to what they claimed was President Mbeki's AIDS denial. The denialist argument was framed by collectivist and historically embedded interpretations of race and identity that were a product of South Africa's colonial and apartheid past. It will be argued that whereas President Mbeki drew on a nationalist and communitarian response to this historical legacy, TAC emerged from an NGO-social movement partnership that deployed global discourses of science, medicine, liberal rights and social justice together with grassroots mobilisation. This globally connected popular struggle for cheaper anti-retroviral (ARV) generic drugs, and for free access to anti-retroviral drugs in the public health system, was in some respects similar to the housing activists' strategies of 'grassroots globalisation' that were discussed in Chapter 4. Like the SDI, PD and SAHPF activists in the preceding chapter, the MSF–TAC alliance forged an NGO-social movement partnership that also had to negotiate complex and contradictory political processes at local, national and global levels.

These global–local struggles for treatment generated new forms of biological and therapeutic citizenship, gendered identities and political subjectivities. In the course of their campaigns, TAC and MSF also had to find ways of dealing with the complex ways in which assumptions about bodily autonomy usually associated with liberal 'rights talk' and biomedicine collided with patriarchal cultural ideas and practices that prevented many women, including many of their own members, from accessing biomedical technologies and interventions (for example, condoms, HIV testing and treatment). The global biomedical paradigm that underpinned TAC's treatment literacy and grassroots mobilisation campaigns also had to address 'local' cultural understandings of misfortune and illness, including beliefs about the occult. In other words, while TAC adopted globally connected biomedical and rights-based approaches to fight the pandemic, they also had to grapple with locally embedded social and cultural obstacles to treatment access. These activist interventions straddled the contradictions and complexities of local, national and global discourses. Science became a key site of contestation, with AIDS statistics becoming a particularly volatile site for speaking about AIDS, race, colonialism and apartheid.

The colour of science in a global age: AIDS, race & (neo)colonialism

AIDS statistics in South Africa have unleashed an extraordinary amount of political heat, controversy and contestation, with the government persistently questioning the reliability of such figures and projections (See Zapiro cartoon p. xv). Matters came to a head in 2001 with the 'leak' to the press of a Medical Research Council (MRC) report which estimated that 'AIDS accounted for about 25% of all deaths in the year 2000 and has become the single biggest cause of death'. The government's initial response to the MRC report was to challenge its findings by claiming that violent death, not AIDS, was the single biggest cause of death. This triggered a major controversy that raged in the media, culminating in the government's concerted efforts to delay the release of the MRC report, while applying considerable pressure on the MRC Board chair to institute a forensic enquiry to uncover the source of the press leak.

The MRC President, Dr Malegapuru Makgoba, was also subjected to pressure to withdraw the report, with government spokespersons claiming that its findings were 'alarmist' and 'inaccurate' (See Zapiro cartoon p. xiv). In response, he stated in 2002 in *MRC News* that the long-term effects of political interference threatened 'the whole national system of innovation in general', while posing 'the greatest threat to the MRC and health research in particular'.[2] Makgoba also reminded his readers of the dangers of the 'Sovietisation of science' and drew attention to Stalin's direct role in ensuring that Lysenko's views dominated Soviet science in the early decades of the twentieth century. In what appeared to be a direct reference to the political interference of President Mbeki and the minister of health in scientific research in South Africa, Dr Makgoba noted:

> Let us also remember what collusion between scientists and the State did for the Nazis, and apartheid South Africa. Finally, let us also remember what happened to science in post-colonial Africa – it has been decimated by uninformed and foolish political decisions and choices. African political leadership should be ashamed of itself in this regard.

[2] *MRC News*, 2002, p. 6.

By the end of 2003, the controversy concerning the MRC Report, dissident science and AIDS statistics seemed to be something of the past.[3] President Mbeki was also no longer publicly supporting the AIDS dissidents, and his Cabinet had committed R12 billion to a national anti-retroviral therapy (ART) programme. However, in February 2004 the stats wars were again in the newspaper headlines with President Mbeki claiming that it was necessary to establish a commission to investigate whether official AIDS mortality figures were accurate or not. Meanwhile, his minister of health, Manto Tshabalala-Msimang, continued claiming in press statements and at conferences that African traditional medicine and a diet of African potatoes, garlic, beetroot and olive were viable alternatives to ARVs, which the president and some senior government officials had earlier claimed were dangerous, toxic, ineffective, too costly and inappropriate for Third World contexts.

One of the possible interpretations of this response from government was that the statistics were perceived to imply that the government was not managing the pandemic effectively, the situation was out of control, and this could have negative impacts in terms of much needed overseas investment. Other possible reasons for this change include discomfort with the findings amongst certain sectors of government and the ruling ANC party who believed that the report reinforced media and popular beliefs and prejudices that AIDS is a 'black disease' concentrated in the rural areas of the former black 'homelands' of KwaZulu-Natal and the Eastern Cape provinces. This racial and geographical profiling of AIDS, it would appear, shaped both state and citizen responses. The questions of race and identity, I argue, lie at the heart of responses to the AIDS pandemic and to AIDS science. The racialised character of these responses was not, however, confined to President Mbeki's inner circle. It has been far more widespread.

In December 2002, the Human Science Research Council (HSRC) released a study that questioned popular perceptions about the racial and geographical distribution of AIDS. A large-scale household survey was conducted to determine the HIV prevalence rates in different provinces, among races, sexes and geographical locations. In an article entitled 'AIDS Survey Shatters Stereotypes', the *Mail and Guardian* reported that 'KwaZulu-Natal has shaken off the tag of having the highest HIV-prevalence rate [and] the Western Cape[4] gets a wake-up call because its HIV prevalence rate of 10.7% is higher than the 8.6% revealed by [MRC] antenatal survey.' The article also noted 'a surprising finding is that the Eastern Cape has the lowest prevalence rate (6.6%).' In contrast to studies that indicated that AIDS prevalence was highest among poor, rural, uneducated black people of the

---

[3] The South African writer and journalist, Rian Malan, attempted to reopen the statistics debate by questioning the accuracy of official statistics on AIDS deaths. He claimed that these figures were grossly overestimated and that existing statistical models were fundamentally flawed. Malan's 'dissident' position was vigorously challenged by TAC activists. See Malan, *Cape Times*, 17 October 2003; *Rolling Stone*, 22 November 2001; *Noseweek*, December 2003; *The Spectator*, 13–20 December 2003; 'Can we Trust Aids Statistics?', *Sunday Times*, 19 October 2003. Responses to Malan included letters from Prof. Ed Rybicki, Department of Molecular and Cell Biology, University of Cape Town, 'Aids Dissent Based on Fallacies', and Nathan Geffen, TAC National Manager, 'Rian Malan Spreads Confusion about AIDS Statistics', both in *Sunday Times*, 2 November 2003.

[4] This historically white and Coloured province was assumed to be the least vulnerable to AIDS prior to the HSRC findings.

former homelands, the HSRC study found that highly mobile urban people in the informal settlements and townships, as well as the middle classes in the suburbs, were most certainly at risk.[5]

Notwithstanding this challenge to AIDS stereotypes and prejudices, the 'cold facts' of AIDS statistics are likely to continue to produce competing interpretations, including those that construct AIDS as a 'black disease'.[6] It is therefore quite conceivable that African nationalists such as President Mbeki interpreted these statistics as evidence of a long colonial and apartheid legacy of scientific racism. In other words, they were read through the colour-coded lens of colonial histories of discrimination and dispossession. For Mbeki and his dissident supporters, such findings were not the product of neutral, rational and universal scientific enquiry, but were understood as the products of historically constructed and politically driven processes embedded in specific histories of colonialism, apartheid and capitalism. He more or less stated this in a speech at the University of Fort Hare in October 2001. Having referred to medical schools as racist institutions where black people were 'reminded of their role as germ carriers', he added,

> thus does it happen that others who consider themselves our leaders take to the streets carrying their placards, to demand that because we are germ carriers, and human beings of a lower order that cannot subject its [sic] passions to reason, we must perforce adopt strange opinions, to save a depraved and diseased people from perishing from self-inflicted disease ... Convinced that we are but natural-born, promiscuous carriers of germs, unique in the world, they proclaim that our continent is doomed to an inevitable mortal end because of our unconquerable devotion to the sin of lust.[7]

In South Africa, the highly politicised dissident debate, 'stats wars' and the numerous cultural obstacles encountered when implementing AIDS prevention programmes have forced scientists, NGOs, AIDS activists and government to acknowledge and respond to local and lay interpretations of AIDS that challenge the scientific truth claims of global biomedicine. These include the blaming of AIDS on witchcraft, as well as a variety of AIDS conspiracies: whites who want to contain black population growth; white doctors who inject patients with AIDS when they go for tests; the CIA and pharmaceutical companies who want to create markets for drugs in Africa; the use of Africans as guinea pigs for scientific experiments with AIDS drugs; beliefs that sex with virgins, including infants, can cure AIDS; and beliefs that anti-retrovirals are dangerously toxic. But perhaps the most daunting problem for AIDS activists and health professionals was the president's

[5] *Mail & Guardian*, 6 December 2002. The HSRC study estimated the overall HIV prevalence in the South African population at 11.4 per cent, or about 4.5 million people. Other estimates put the figure at between 5 and 7 million.

[6] Although the HSRC 2002 AIDS prevalence report found that all races were at risk, Africans had the highest incidence rate with 18.4 per cent. Whites and Coloureds were around 6 per cent and Indians 1.8 per cent. The 6 per cent rate for whites was up from 2 per cent in 2000, at a time when the white population was perceived to be eight years behind the prevalence in the African population (M. Colvin *et al.*, 2000, cited in T. Marcus, 'Kissing the Cobra: Sexuality and High Risk in a Generalised Epidemic – a Case Study', paper presented for the conference 'AIDS in Context', University of the Witwatersrand, Johannesburg, March 2001).

[7] *Mail & Guardian*, 'Mbeki in Bizarre AIDS Outburst', 26 October 2001. Cited in Deborah Posel's chapter on AIDS in Steven Robins and Nick Shephard (eds) *New South African Keywords* (in press).

initial flirtation with AIDS dissident theories and the implications this had in terms of attempts to establish AIDS treatment programmes. The President's position, along with a plethora of popularly held 'AIDS myths' and the stigma and shame associated with AIDS, contributed towards defensive responses and AIDS denial amongst both the general population as well as within the president's inner circle of policymakers and politicians. What are the implications of all this for contemporary debates on the role of NGOs and social movements in mediating science and citizenship in a globalising world?

Mediating science: the role of NGOs and social movements

The AIDS pandemic in South Africa raises a number of troubling dilemmas for NGO and social movement attempts to globalise and democratise science and biomedicine, especially in the Third World. Given the relative weakness of African states and the extremely thin spread of scientific knowledge and institutions, what can 'citizen science', popular epidemiology, ethnoscience and indigenous knowledge do to deal with a lethal pandemic such as AIDS? Or would state legitimisation of these public knowledges not further undermine already weak scientific institutions and biomedical knowledge regimes? What does 'citizen science' mean in contexts where contestation between the public's and experts' forms of knowledge and science threatens to undermine biomedical scientific authority and AIDS interventions that could potentially save lives? What about contexts where contestation over AIDS science becomes highly politicised because governments are distrustful of the autonomy of the scientific establishment, or where indigenous knowledge and local solutions are reified as part of cultural nationalist ideologies and programmes? What about situations where people's own knowledge and practices result in AIDS denial, violence and oppression – as when, for instance, the South African AIDS counsellor Gugu Dlamini revealed her HIV-positive status to rural villagers, who responded by killing her for bringing shame and disease to her community?

This case study explores notions such as the 'democratisation of science' for NGOs and social movements located within the epicentre of the worst public health hazard in Africa's history. It focuses on the opportunities and constraints that exist for NGOs and social movements to create favourable conditions for mediation and negotiation between various experts and publics, given this state of emergency (see Leach *et al.* 2005). The AIDS pandemic raises particularly difficult questions concerning the role of these actors in facilitating deliberative and inclusionary processes in scientific domains: Who is to be invited into what fora? What do these deliberative processes mean in contexts where scientific authority is distrusted both by powerful individuals within the state, and by large sections of the public?

By focusing on the responses and strategies of government, AIDS activists and civil society organisations such as TAC, it is possible to begin to address some of these questions. This case study investigates TAC's creative engagement with a global community of experts – scientists, lawyers, doctors, NGOs and so on – as well as its grassroots constituencies, and examines the opportunities and limits that framed TAC's interactions within these global–local spaces.

The 'AIDS dissident debate' in South Africa is not merely academic. For example, certain lay knowledges and alternative, fringe, scientific perspectives (AIDS dissident science) have translated into support for AIDS myths and conspiracy theories that have, according to AIDS activists and health professionals, had a devastating impact on public health interventions, directly contributing to the loss of tens of thousands of lives. Some AIDS activists blamed dissidents and AIDS denialists within government for failing to provide ARV treatment, and thereby contributing towards 600 AIDS deaths each day. Dr Costa Gazi of the Pan Africanist Congress (PAC) went as far as claiming that this shortcoming constituted a crime against humanity and complicity in genocide. The self-identified HIV-positive Justice Edwin Cameron, of the Supreme Court of Appeal, ultimately saw the triumph of apartheid thinking in the deniers:

> We have a crisis of AIDS in our country. On the one hand that crisis is one of illness and suffering and dying – dying on a larger scale and in conspicuously different patterns from before; on a scale globally that dwarfs any disease or epidemic the world has known for more than six centuries. On the other hand that crisis is one of leadership and management … The most fundamental crisis in the AIDS epidemic is our nation's struggle to identify and confront and act on the truth about AIDS. … The denial of AIDS represents the ultimate relic of apartheid's racially imposed consciousness, and the deniers achieve the ultimate victory of the apartheid mindset.[8]

While the dissident debate raged on, TAC activists, health professionals and the trade unions took to the streets and the courts in the struggle for AIDS treatment based on citizens' constitutionally-enshrined rights to health care. Zapiro,[9] the best known of South Africa's political cartoonists, graphically captured this by depicting the president as playing the dissident fiddle while Rome was burning (See Zapiro cartoon p. xv). In the face of relentless criticism of the President's pro-dissident stance, his spokespersons and supporters argued against the guild-like exclusivism of the scientific community and insisted upon the democratic right of the President to participate in debates on AIDS science. AIDS activists and health professionals made the counter-argument that the President's role in the debate was undermining public health institutions and the scientific authority and autonomy of experts, scientists and health professionals. While this case of high-level political interference in the scientific arena may appear extreme and exceptional, it nonetheless draws attention to more general questions relating to science, medicine, politics and citizenship in an age of globalisation.

Nationalist solidarities versus cosmopolitan science

AIDS is a global disease that has devastated communities struggling under the burdens of poverty, inequality, economic crisis and war (Shoepf 2001). AIDS is

---

8   This quote is from Judge Edwin Cameron's speech delivered at the launch of photographer Gideon Mendel's book, *A Broken Landscape*, at the South African National Gallery, Cape Town, Saturday 13 April 2002.

9   Zapiro's real name is Jonathan Shapiro.

also 'an epidemic of signification' (Treichler 1999) and responses to it have been unrelentingly moralising and stigmatising. In Africa, this 'geography of blame' (Farmer 1992) has contributed towards racist representations of African sexualities as diseased, dangerous, promiscuous and uncontrollable. This in turn has triggered defensive (nationalist) reactions that draw on dissident AIDS science, conspiracy theories and AIDS denial among African politicians, officials, intellectuals and journalists.

Representational politics have plagued AIDS debates and interventions in South Africa. These issues have had a profound impact upon the ways in which civil society and the state responded to the pandemic. Virtually every aspect of the pandemic – from AIDS statistics, to theories about the causal link between HIV and AIDS, to studies on AIDS drug therapy – led to contestation between government on the one side, and AIDS activists, scientists, health professionals and the media on the other. Given perceptions that AIDS fuels racist representations of Africans, it was perhaps not surprising that responses from President Mbeki took such a defensive turn.

The AIDS dissident debate in South Africa can be narrated from a variety of angles. It can be told as a story of how a small but powerful policy network was built around President Mbeki, and how this 'inner circle' was able to shape the direction of AIDS policy in South Africa. It is also the story of the Treatment Action Campaign (TAC) and a highly organised and globally connected community of scientists, health professionals, and civil society organisations who contested this dissident line. By November 2002, after three years of mass mobilisation, court cases, civil disobedience campaigns and demonstrations calling for AIDS treatment, the dissidents were on the retreat and ARV treatment was in sight. In August 2003 the Cabinet announced that it had decided to go ahead with a national ARV programme. But how and why did South Africa follow this tortuous path?

It was only in the late 1980s that AIDS in South Africa began to be acknowledged as a serious public health problem. Prior to this it was widely perceived to be a North American 'gay disease', with San Francisco and New York at its centres. It took almost a decade for the seriousness of the AIDS pandemic to filter into the consciousness of South African citizens, the media and policymakers. By the time of the World AIDS Conference in Durban in July 2000, most South Africans were aware that the country was in the midst of an epidemic of catastrophic proportions.

This conference also exposed the international AIDS community to the deep rift between mainstream AIDS scientists and government supporters of the AIDS dissidents. Versions of the dissident view were articulated by President Mbeki and senior ANC figures such as the late Parks Mankahlana and Peter Mokaba, both of whom are believed to have died of AIDS.[10] In a press statement reported in the *Mail & Guardian* newspaper on 19 April 2002, a few months before his death, Mokaba, the ANC chief electoral officer, presented the AIDS dissident position in

---

[10]   It is unclear how far these views were shared within the top echelons of the ANC government. There are nonetheless indications that there was considerable disagreement with Mbeki's stance, even within his cabinet. The strongest internal criticism came from the ANC's Tripartite Alliance partners, the South African Communist Party (SACP) and the Congress of South African Trade Unions (COSATU).

the following terms:

> The story that HIV causes AIDS is being promoted through lies, pseudo-science, violence, terrorism and deception … We are urged to abandon science and adopt the religion of super-stition that HIV exists and that it causes AIDS. We refuse to be agents for using our people as guinea pigs and have a responsibility to defeat the intended genocide and dehumanisation of the African family and society.[11]

This line of argument, which was elaborated in detail by South African and inter-national dissidents, was mercilessly challenged and lampooned by cartoonists and journalists. Its critics also included academics, opposition parties, AIDS activists and health professionals. Yet despite a considerable challenge to the dissident view, even within the ruling party, it nonetheless came to represent the official gov-ernment position on AIDS. This culminated in President Mbeki's establishment of the President's Select Advisory Panel of AIDS experts comprising an equal weight-ing of 'establishment scientists' and AIDS dissidents (See Zapiro cartoon p. xiv).

In March 2002 a controversial AIDS dissident document was posted on the ANC website. Its full title was *Castro Hlongwane, Caravans, Cats, Geese, Foot & Mouth and Statistics: HIV/AIDS and the Struggle for the Humanisation of the African.*[12] The document was subjected to intense criticism and ridicule from AIDS activists and the media, who portrayed it as an endorsement of President Mbeki's eccentric views. It quoted numerous scientific studies and journalistic forays questioning 'mainstream' AIDS science.[13] Throughout, the author(s) referred to the 'omnipotent apparatus' that sought to bring about the dehumanisation of the African family and humiliate 'our people' (that is Africans). Citing numerous newspaper articles and scientific findings, the *Castro Hlongwane* document blamed AIDS drugs and phar-maceutical companies for 'the medicalisation of poverty' and for systematically destroying the immune systems of Africans. The posting also claimed that 'for the omnipotent apparatus [which includes the media, the medical establishment and drug companies] the most important thing is the marketing of the anti-retroviral drugs.' It concluded with the following statement:

> No longer will the Africans accept as the unalterable truth that they are a dependent people that emanates from and inhabits a continent shrouded in a terrible darkness of destructive superstition, driven and sustained by ignorance, hunger and underdevelopment, and that is

---

[11] Cited in Gitay, J. 'Rhetoric, Politics, Science, Medicine: The South African HIV/AIDS Controversy' (unpublished paper, Centre for African Studies, University of Cape Town, 18 September 2002), p. 2.

[12] The *Castro Hlongwane* document was allegedly posted on the ANC website by Peter Mokaba and is a lengthy exposition of the dissident position. The anonymous author, for example, 'rejects as baseless and self-serving the assertion that millions of our people are HIV positive … It therefore rejects the sugges-tion that the challenge of AIDS in our country can be solved by resort to anti-retroviral drugs … It rejects the assertion that, among the nations, we have the highest incidence of HIV infection and AIDS deaths, caused by sexual immorality of our people.' The author goes on to claim in Chapter VI, 'We do not know how many of our people have died [because scientists and doctors] at Chris Hani Baragwanath Hospital, conducted experiments on our people or "treated" them [with anti-retrovirals], relying on dangerously tendentious results of clinical [trials] sponsored by the pharmaceutical companies.'

[13] The document also included numerous literary, journalistic and academic citations ranging from Adam Hochschild's *King Leopold's Ghost* (1998), Herbert Marcuse's *Eros & Civilisation* (1970), Paul Farmer's *AIDS and Accusation* (1993) and Angela Davis's *Women, Race and Class*, to a smattering of quotes from a diverse group of writers such as Henry Louis Gates, Jr., W.B. Yeats, Mark Twain, Jeffrey Sachs, John le Carré, Sun Tzu and many others.

victim to a self-inflicted "disease" called HIV/AIDS. *For centuries we have carried the burden of the crimes and falsities of 'scientific' Eurocentrism, its dogmas imposed upon our being as brands of a definitive, 'universal' truth. Against this, we have, in struggle, made the statement to which we will remain loyal – that we are human and African!* (italics in original)

Although officially the ANC attempted to distance itself from the document in response to fierce general criticism, it became evident that the document's focus on the legacies of colonialism, underdevelopment, poverty, the Eurocentrism of science and racist representations of Africans as a 'diseased Other' appealed to a small group of African nationalists within the ANC leadership. *Castro Hlongwane* reads as an African nationalist defence of the AIDS dissident position in the face of what its authors claimed was a racist representation of AIDS as a 'black disease' associated with sexual promiscuity and the inability of Africans to control their sexual appetites. More generally, racist narratives about the sexually promiscuous black African fuelled Mokaba and Mbeki's African nationalist response. This may help explain support for their dissident ideas.

TAC adopted a very different approach by seeking to destigmatise and depathologise African sexualities. For instance, in Jack Lewis's much acclaimed documentary film on TAC, entitled *Aluta Continua*, the key male and female characters, both of whom are black HIV-positive AIDS activists, consciously seek to affirm black African sexualities. They state that there is nothing to be ashamed about in having multiple partners, and it is quite normal and acceptable as long as safe sex is practised. This sexual permissiveness, together with TAC's open support for gay and lesbian sexual rights, led to attempts by some senior ANC politicians to discredit TAC by claiming that its hidden agenda, apart from being a front for 'Big Pharma,' was to introduce liberal ideas about sexuality that were in line with those held by the international gay and lesbian movement.

Historically, Third World nationalist intellectuals have been very active in challenging what they have perceived as western ethnocentrism, especially when it comes to matters of culture, women and the family, sexuality, spirituality, religion, and so on. Partha Chatterjee (1993) has shown how anti-colonial nationalists in India produced their own domain of sovereignty within colonial society before beginning their political battle with the imperial power. This involved staking out an autonomous spiritual sphere represented by religion, caste, women and the family and peasants. Not surprisingly, African nationalists, like their Indian counterparts, generated their own gendered nationalisms that accepted the western culture of the state, while simultaneously carving out sovereignty in the domain of African culture, and African women and the family. However, AIDS threatens the integrity of this domain of sovereignty by appearing morally to condemn African male sexualities, as well as declaring the failure of the African family to live up to the western nuclear family ideal. It is resistance to this perceived moral and cultural onslaught that animates the African nationalist response to AIDS. Just as the dissident view attributed AIDS to African poverty and disease reproduced through western racism, colonial conquest, capitalism and underdevelopment, it also challenged attempts to attribute the African AIDS pandemic to dysfunctional sexualities and family structures.

Rhetoric, rights and scientific relativism

While active dissident support may have been limited to a relatively small circle of intellectuals, journalists and politicians, this position resonated with, and possibly gave credibility to, popular forms of AIDS denial and alternative and traditional explanations for AIDS and illness. This popular contestation of establishment AIDS science is hardly surprising given that many South Africans, like citizens in Europe and North America, are suspicious of expertise from which they have always been excluded. As a result, HIV/AIDS has been assimilated into a variety of popular epistemologies and local ways of making sense of disease and misfortune, for example, witchcraft and Christianity.[14]

Following two years of confusing mixed messages, in 2002 President Mbeki appeared to distance himself from the dissidents, claiming that public perception of the government's support for the dissidents reflected a 'failure of communication on our side'.[15] But was this simply 'a failure of communication'? Responding to President Mbeki's forays into AIDS science, Joshua Gitay concludes that politicians, who 'lack scientific tools', should not be allowed to base their health policies on rhetoric, but should instead follow the consensus of the health sciences: the experts' translation of the scientific data (Gitay 2002: 25). In support, he quotes approvingly from Sulcas and Gordin, who argue that *'HIV/AIDS is not a freedom of speech issue. It is about scientifically verifiable facts. There are findings that, after testing, an overwhelming number of scientists consider accurate'* (emphasis added).[16]

While AIDS activists and the media described the positions of Mbeki and Mokaba as irrational, politically-motivated, and incompatible with western science, it would appear that the dissidents were insisting on their democratic right to criticise the science establishment. They did this by drawing attention to their alternative science. ANC spokespersons attempted to justify this high-level government intervention by referring to it as an expression of freedom of thought: a matter of rights. They described Mbeki as a latter-day Galileo burned at the stake by the media for refusing to conform to scientific orthodoxy. Calls for Mbeki to withdraw from the debate were described as attempts by the 'scientific guild' to shut down and stifle debate on questionable scientific findings. Mbeki's spokespersons also described his interventions as an attempt to open up what was perceived to be a narrowly technical, biomedical framing of the AIDS pandemic that ignored conditions of poverty and underdevelopment. Whereas much of this critique of the biomedical paradigm would have sat comfortably with most left-leaning South African AIDS and public health activists, the questioning of the link between the HI virus and AIDS was what went beyond the pale. It was this strand of the dissident critique that was perceived to be discontinuous with the global consensus

---

[14] I am grateful to Renee Fox (personal communication) for insightful e-mail discussions on the relationship between 'dissident' views and 'popular' religious and spiritual beliefs about illness and disease derived from her work with *Médecins Sans Frontières* in Khayelitsha, Cape Town, and other parts of the world.

[15] *Cape Times*, 25 April 2002.

[16] A. Sulcas, J. Gordin, *Sunday Independent*, 23 April 2000.

on AIDS science. Notwithstanding the status of the president as the leader of the ANC, a former national liberation movement that continues to command deep loyalty from the vast majority of South Africans, his deployment of race and nationalist rhetoric in his challenge to mainstream AIDS science appeared to fail to win widespread support from within his own party, the trade union movement and the broader public. Yet, along with his health minister's persistent promotion of dietary alternatives to ARVs, the president's interventions had an undeniably adverse impact on public health efforts to expand treatment access. By 2008 only 371,731 (42%) of an estimated 889,000 people who needed treatment, were receiving ARVs through the public health sector.[17] AIDS activists and public health professionals blamed this slow pace on lack of political will and leadership from the president down.

Science, conspiracies and biomedical citizenship

Given the history of South Africa, it is perhaps not surprising that race and cultural identity came to assume such a central place in public discourses on AIDS. By the time AIDS began to take such a visible toll on South Africa, the country had barely surfaced from apartheid, a political system characterised by extreme forms of social and economic inequalities and ideological domination that systematically denigrated and dehumanised black people. As a result of this history, as well as colonial legacies of deep distrust of western science and modernisation policies,[18] President Mbeki was able to make the claim that AIDS was being interpreted through a profoundly racialised (and racist) lens: African sexualities are dysfunctional, and Africans are to blame for their morally irresponsible and destructive sexual behaviour. The president no doubt felt compelled to challenge these racist readings of black bodies and sexualities, as did many other African nationalists. It would seem that AIDS had become a Rorschach, an ideological screen upon which a range of fears and fantasies could be projected. Mbeki's response suggests that he believed that there was a widespread view that it was the socially irresponsible, excessive and immoral sexual practices of Africans that was the root cause of the spread of the AIDS pandemic: the victim is to blame. Although HIV/AIDS exists amongst white, middle-class heterosexual communities throughout the world, the stigma of its early associations with homosexuals, bisexuals, blacks, sex workers and drug users has continued to stick. This troubling genealogy of the disease continues to shape the AIDS debate in South Africa. It explains the intense sense of shame associated with AIDS as well as the attraction of dissident AIDS science and nationalist views, especially amongst young, educated black South Africans. A TAC activist spoke of a limited degree of support for Mbeki's dissident views amongst intellectuals and educated township youth, while in the

---

[17] www.tac.org.za/community/keystatistics

[18] Africa has a long colonial legacy of contestation over 'scientific' versus 'local' knowledge about environmental degradation relating to pastoralism, forest management, and soil and water conservation. Africans' distrust of 'western science' and 'development' often resulted in fierce resistance to colonial cattle culling policies that were justified on the basis of foot and mouth disease or overstocking. In many cases such grievances concerning colonial development and conservation interventions contributed towards swelling the ranks of the liberation movements and advanced the cause of anti-colonial struggles.

rural areas she encountered more widespread AIDS denial and myths. It appeared that while TAC may have won the battle for ARV treatment, and in the process mobilised thousands of people living with AIDS, it had not yet won the war against misinformation, fear, denial, silence and shame. The contestation and politicisation of AIDS science and ARVs continued, as did numerous AIDS conspiracies and controversies.

In January 2005 TAC's Zackie Achmat argued in a newspaper article that 'science, or truth, does not modify itself for our ideological wishes' (*Mail & Guardian*, 21 January 2005). Achmat is also known to express his utter disdain for post-structuralist deconstruction, especially when it comes to issues relating to AIDS. This brand of deeply held 'scientific positivism', perhaps verging on 'techno-fundamentalism', emerged in the context of ongoing contestation about a variety of aspects relating to AIDS science, ARVs and so on. These debates reinforced the beliefs of many South African citizens that science was indeed highly politicised and ideological. Whereas science is usually portrayed in the formal education system as an apolitical, technical and objective enterprise, the persistent AIDS controversies circulating in the mass media fundamentally questioned this assumption. One of the unintended consequences of this scientific contestation was that many South Africans became increasingly aware of the complex relationship between science, politics and ideology, for instance in terms of the ideological shaping of research, the (mis)use of scientific results, control over funding, and the use of science-as-ideology.

This growing public recognition of the politicised, ideological and instrumental character of AIDS science is part of a broader worldwide phenomenon of citizen distrust of science and expertise. It is also related to increasing calls for citizen participation in scientific juries and the adjudication of scientific knowledge (Beck 1992; Epstein 1996; Leach, Scoones and Wynne 2004). Distrust in scientific authority has also found expression in Nigeria, where a group of Islamic clerics in the northern state of Kano led an immunisation boycott, claiming that the polio vaccine was part of a US-led plot to render Muslims infertile or infect them with the HI virus (*Associated Press*, 13 January 2005). Similarly, a telephone survey conducted by RAND Corporation and Oregon State University indicated that a significant number of African Americans surveyed believed that US government scientists created HIV to eradicate or control African–American populations (*Kaiser Daily HIV/AIDS Report*, 2 February 2005). This distrust of science and medicine is of course not confined to Africa. As Melissa Leach (2005) has shown, citizen mobilisation against the British Health Department's compulsory MMR vaccinations of children revealed similar levels of citizen distrust of science and medicine. A number of UK parents recently challenged the safety of MMR, arguing that there is a direct link between MMR vaccinations and forms of childhood autism their children suffer. They also claimed that scientists were being co-opted by the pharmaceutical companies and the state to provide scientific evidence supporting the government's vaccination programmes. All this conspiracy talk and distrust of mainstream science and the medical industry sounds quite familiar to South Africans, where contestation of orthodox AIDS science and treatment technologies continues to be reported in the media. It also explains the urgency with which Zackie Achmat sought to combat these forms of popular scientific relativism by asserting that scientific truth should not be sacrificed in the name of political ideology.

Former president Mandela also attempted to contain this 'confusion' by publicly stating that his son had died of AIDS. It was part of his explicitly stated effort to get South Africans to treat AIDS as an ordinary treatable and manageable chronic illness like tuberculosis (TB), cancer or diabetes. It was also an attempt to assert the scientific reality of HIV/AIDS as the leading cause of death in South Africa in the face of persistent AIDS denial. Mandela's statement was immediately challenged by the United States-based AIDS dissident David Rasnick, who claimed that it was antiretroviral (ARV) drugs, not AIDS, that had killed Makgatho Mandela (*Sunday Times*, 16 January 2005).

Rasnick was not alone in claiming that ARVs were toxic. For example, the national Health Minister Manto Tshabalala-Msimang, the South African Traditional Healers Organisation (THO), the Mattias Rath Foundation, the writer and journalist Rian Malan, and an anonymous author on the ANC website all questioned TAC's credentials and motivations for lobbying for ARV treatment. THO and Rath Foundation were affiliates of the Treatment Information Group, an organisation that accused TAC of being the salespersons of the pharmaceutical industry, and claimed that Dr Rath's multinutrients could reduce the risk of developing AIDS by 50 per cent. These organisations also claimed that TAC was exaggerating AIDS statistics, and using Africans as guinea pigs for the marketing of toxic AIDS drugs (*Mail & Guardian*, 24 December 2004). What these coordinated attacks revealed was the emergence of a network that implicitly aligned itself with President Mbeki and AIDS dissident scientists such as David Rasnick and Peter Duesberg and their supporters. These South African and US dissidents claimed that there was clandestine collusion between AIDS activists, scientists and the pharmaceutical industry. They suggested that these powerful networks and political influences controlled scientific research in order to serve the business interests of 'Big Pharma'. Notwithstanding all this conspiracy talk, the South African Government facilitated the pharmaceutical giant Aspen's programme for the large-scale manufacture of ARVs in Port Elizabeth.

Despite the decision by government to establish a national ARV programme, the health minister and her supporters claimed that drug companies, in collusion with scientists, were undermining the credibility of natural and traditional medicines. Her response was to promote a diet of virgin olive oil, onions, the African potato and garlic, which she claimed could boost the immune systems of AIDS sufferers. She also claimed that HIV-positive citizens should be given the right to choose their own treatment, be it traditional and alternative medicines or ARVs. Activists, scientists and public health professionals insisted that rigorous scientific testing ought to determine the range of treatment options; biomedical citizenship, in other words, required that patients had scientific information at their disposal so that they could make reasonable decisions about their health.

By 2008, the debate on the efficacy and safety of ARVs and traditional medicines for AIDS patients was far from resolved. Meanwhile, the South African government had allowed health care centres to provide complementary and traditional medicines to HIV-positive patients. This decision was based on department of health estimates that up to 70 per cent of South Africans consult traditional healers. However, South African doctors and scientists remained sceptical about claims concerning the benefits of herbal and traditional medicines for AIDS patients, especially those on ARV therapy (*Sunday Independent*, 30 January 2005). Their argument, like the position of TAC's Zackie Achmat, was that traditional medicines had to be scientifically tested. As Achmat put, it was necessary to modernise traditional healing through regulation and rigorous testing of the efficacy and safety of these medicines.

For TAC activists the Rath Foundation's promotion of conspiracy theories and alternative and traditional remedies for HIV/AIDS had life and death consequences. From this perspective there was no room for cultural or scientific relativism, and TAC's lawyers resorted to legal challenges and hard-nosed scientific evidence to challenge the claims of the Minister of Health, the Rath Foundation and the Traditional Healers Organisation.

TAC lawyers and activists were not alone in perceiving scientific relativism as a potential threat to human lives. Bruno Latour, the doyen of Science Studies, questioned his own role in promoting the idea that political networks comprising scientists, research institutes, universities, industry and funding agencies collude in ways that influence the construction of scientific facts. Latour and his colleagues also devoted their intellectual careers towards trying to demonstrate the absence of scientific certainty inherent in the construction of facts. Latour's path-breaking work demonstrated the influence of 'extra-scientific' factors emanating from beyond the confines of the laboratory. He argued that the politics of research funding, scientific networks, research committees and the peer-reviewed journal system all played a decisive role in maintaining or 'closing down' scientific controversies and debates. Scientific truth, Latour had argued, was established through the networks, funding circuits and power plays that scientists were obliged to participate in.

Latour (2005) has reflected on the unintended consequences of his earlier writings on the social construction of scientific facts as possibly being an awful mistake. He illustrates his concern with the example of Mr. Lutz, a conservative US Republican strategist, who advises his clients that they 'need to continue to make the lack of scientific certainty [about global warming] the primary issue'. While Latour tells us that his project has been to 'emancipate the public from prematurely naturalised objectified facts', this Republican strategist was using the same approach to assist conservative and ecologically unfriendly corporate interests to sustain scientific controversy in the name of profit margins. For Latour this kind of scenario raises serious political, ethical and scientific dilemmas.

The Rath Foundation has drawn on similar strategies to maintain scientific uncertainty about key aspects of AIDS science. This occurred despite the fact that the AIDS dissident position was dismissed and discredited in mainstream scientific circles in Europe and North America as early as the mid-1980s. South Africa's dissidents also sought to frame the AIDS debate within anti-racist and anti-colonial discourses that blame the spread of the pandemic in Africa on structural conditions of racism, poverty and underdevelopment. While many South African public health professionals acknowledge the need to understand the impact of poverty and inequality in driving the pandemic in Africa, they stress the link between HIV and AIDS and the fact that AIDS in Africa is primarily a heterosexually transmitted disease. They argue that HIV/AIDS is a product of human agency as well as structural conditions of poverty and inequality. TAC activists and public health experts thus argue that part of the task of AIDS activism is to create the conditions for production of 'responsibilised citizens' (See Chapter 6).

It is not clear to what degree the Rath Foundation's conspiracy theories about the hidden links between AIDS science, medicine and the pharmaceutical industry resonated with the views of ordinary South Africans. But it is clear that TAC took Rath's organisation sufficiently seriously to litigate against the foundation's misinformation campaigns and to publicly refute Rath's claims that ARVs were toxic and that his multivitamins were a better remedy for HIV/AIDS. It would seem that Rath's conspiracy theories resonate with growing global scepticism and distrust of science and the multi-billion dollar drug industry. It is within this highly politicised context of ongoing scientific controversies and contestations of mainstream AIDS science that TAC launched its litigation strategies, treatment literacy and grassroots mobilisation campaigns. Addressing questions of AIDS science, scientific authority and biomedical citizenship became a central task for TAC activists.

For those HIV-positive, unemployed and working-class black mothers who joined TAC, AIDS denial and dissident and conspiracy theories did not resonate with their all-too-real experiences of contracting the virus from HIV-positive men and losing children to AIDS, a tragedy that they believed could be averted through prevention of mother-to-child-transmission (PMTCT) programmes. For example, V, a young black female TAC volunteer, tells the story of how, following the trauma of rape by an uncle who later committed suicide, she was diagnosed with AIDS, hospitalised and told that she 'must wait for my day of death'. V eventually joined TAC and received ART. For V, TAC literally saved her life, 'Now I can stay alive for a long time. I have my whole life'. The organisation became the family that she lost when she was diagnosed HIV-positive:

> I started the medicine [ART] and I am happy now because my immune system is picking up. So I tell the youngsters they must wake up and fight HIV … TAC has helped me a lot. Before I was scared to go on TV or newspaper, but now I am not, because they give me a lot of support … Mandla and Zackie are like my brother and my father … They are not big guys – they are coming down to us

V's account of her confrontation with AIDS and the spectre of death suggests why the abstract and ideological language of cultural nationalism and conspiracies did not resonate for her. It also draws attention to the experiential dimensions of belonging that TAC is able to provide for HIV-positive people who, once they reveal their HIV status, are often exposed to stigma and rejection from their families and communities. Such trauma highlights the limits of ideological mobilisation in terms of shaping people's understanding of their identities, subjectivities and their place in the world. For TAC activists living openly with AIDS, abstract denialist ideologies, nationalisms or 'imagined communities' cannot easily be conjured up in the absence of experientially based understandings and social realities. However, these abstract ideologies may indeed appeal to those living beyond the sphere of influence of the broad church of AIDS activism.

The following section provides a brief history of TAC in order to reveal how this globally connected social movement was able to mediate ideas about biomedicine and rights as well as catalyse and mobilise a powerful sense of community belonging and identity formation amongst its members. It also provides the historical context for the following chapter, which examines how belonging to TAC and getting on to treatment programmes can contribute to profound transformations in subjectivity that result from illness and treatment experiences, what I refer to in Chapter 6 as the passage from 'near death' to 'new life'.

Treatment Action Campaign (TAC): mediating rights and new subjectivities

TAC was established on 10 December 1998, International Human Rights Day, when a group of about fifteen people protested on the steps of St George's Cathedral in Cape Town to demand medical treatment for people living with the virus that causes AIDS. By the end of the day, the protestors had collected over a thousand signatures calling on the government to develop a treatment plan for all people living with HIV.[19]

TAC's membership has grown dramatically over the past few years. The rank-and-file comprises mainly young urban Africans with secondary schooling. However, the organisation has also managed to attract health professionals and university students. The international face of the organisation is Zackie Achmat, a forty-something Muslim former anti-apartheid and gay activist. He is also a law graduate and an openly HIV-positive person. Until recently Achmat had made it known publicly that he refused to take ART until it was available in the public health sector. Other TAC leaders include African men and women who joined TAC as volunteers and moved into leadership positions over time. The majority of the volunteers are young African women, many of them HIV-positive.

When TAC was founded, it was generally assumed that anti-AIDS drugs were beyond the reach of developing countries, condemning 90 per cent of the world's HIV-positive population to a painful and inevitable death. While TAC's main objective has been to lobby and pressurise the South African government to provide AIDS treatment, it has increasingly addressed a much wider range of issues. These have included tackling the global pharmaceutical industry in the media, the courts and the streets; fighting violence and discrimination against HIV-positive people, gay, lesbian citizens and women; challenging AIDS dissident science; and

---

[19]   For a detailed account of the early history of TAC and its campaign for MTCT prevention programme, see *Treatment Action: An Overview, 1998–2001*, p. 2 in www.tac.org.za.

taking the government to court for refusing to provide MTCT programmes in public health facilities.[20] During these campaigns, TAC mobilised within working-class black communities and the trade union movement, and used a variety of methods to pressurise the global pharmaceutical industry and the South African government to provide cheap ARVs. These modes of mobilisation created the political space for the articulation of new forms of health/biological citizenship linked to attempts to democratise science in post-apartheid South Africa.

Soon after its establishment, in 1998 TAC, together with the South African government, became embroiled in a lengthy legal battle with international pharmaceutical companies over AIDS drug patents and the importation of cheap generics to treat millions of HIV-positive poor people in developing countries. As a result of highly successful global and national media campaigns, TAC managed to convince international public opinion, and the Pharmaceutical Manufacturers' Association (PMA), that it was moral and just for drug companies to bring down their prices and allow developing countries to manufacture generics. In the face of international public opinion in favour of TAC, PMA withdrew their case – no doubt influenced by the costs of adverse publicity that corporate greed was responsible for millions of deaths in Africa.

Despite TAC's highly successful global networking, much of TAC's energy was devoted to more local matters: mobilising poor and working-class communities, using the courts to compel the ministry of health to provide ARVs at public facilities, and campaigning to protect the autonomy of scientific institutions from government interference. Although grassroots mobilisation was primarily in black African working-class areas, TAC's organisational structure and support networks crossed race, class, ethnic, occupational and educational lines.

TAC volunteers were involved in AIDS awareness and treatment literacy campaigns. In addition, TAC disseminated reports, scientific studies, website documents (see Wasserman 2003)[21] and media briefs refuting government claims that ARV treatment was dangerously toxic, ineffective, too costly, and could not be implemented due to infrastructure and logistical problems such as inadequate management structures, shortages of trained staff and so on. The organisation also came out in strong support of doctors, hospital superintendents, medical researchers and the MRC who, by virtue of their report findings or provision of ARV treatment, found themselves on the wrong side of government, and subject to high-level political interference and intimidation.

AIDS activism and 'globalisation from below'
TAC's mode of activism could be described as grassroots globalisation or 'globalisation from below' (Appadurai 2002 a and b). Following the precedent of the

[20] In May 2008, TAC, MSF and the AIDS Law Project became centrally involved in advocating for the rights of thousands of refugees who were expelled from townships during waves of xenophobic violence that spreads across the country. In July 2008, Zackie Achmat launched the Social Justice Coalition to fight poverty, disease, violence, crime and substance abuse in poor communities. However, HIV/AIDS remains at the centre of TAC's campaigns.

[21] Wasserman has a chapter on TAC and the Internet's potential for civil society groups in South Africa.

divestment campaigns of the anti-apartheid struggle, TAC activism straddled local, national and global spaces in the course of struggles for access to cheaper AIDS drugs. This was done through the courts, the Internet, the media and by networking with South African and international civil society organisations. Widely publicised acts of 'civil disobedience' also provided TAC with visibility within a globally connected post-apartheid public sphere. By concentrating on access to ARV treatments for working-class and poor people, TAC was participating in a class-based politics that departed significantly from the cultural nationalist/identity politics promoted by the new ruling elite of Mbeki and Mokaba. It was not coincidental that COSATU, having lost thousands of workers to the pandemic, readily joined the TAC campaign.

The 'Christopher Moraka Defiance Campaign' was perhaps a defining moment in TAC's pro-poor political mobilisation around AIDS. It began in July 2000, after HIV-positive TAC volunteer Christopher Moraka died, suffering from severe thrush. TAC's spokespersons claimed that the drug fluconazole could have eased his pain and prolonged his life, but it was not available on the public health system because it was too expensive. In October 2000, in response to Moraka's death, TAC's Zackie Achmat visited Thailand where he bought 5,000 capsules of a cheap generic fluconazole. When TAC announced Achmat's mission in a press conference the international public outcry against the pharmaceutical giant Pfizer intensified as it became clear how inflated were the prices of name-brand medications; no charges were brought against Achmat, and the drugs were successfully prescribed to South African patients. By March 2001, Pfizer had made its drugs available free of charge to state clinics.

This David and Goliath narrative of TAC's successful challenge to the global pharmaceutical giants captured the imagination of the international community and catapulted TAC into the global arena. Preparation for the court case also consolidated TAC's ties with international NGOs such as Oxfam, *Médecins Sans Frontières*, the European Coalition of Positive People, Health Gap, and Ralph Nader's Consumer Technology Project in the United States. It seemed as if this was indeed a glimpse into what a progressive global civil society could look like.

TAC activists nevertheless stressed that grassroots mobilisation was the key to their success. This was done through AIDS awareness and treatment literacy campaigns in schools, factories, community centres, churches, *shebeens* (informal drinking places), and through door-to-door visits in the African townships. By far the majority of TAC volunteers were poor and unemployed African women, many of them HIV-positive mothers desperate to gain access life-saving drugs for themselves and their children.

TAC was also able to rely on support from middle-class business professionals, health professionals, scientists, the media, and ordinary South African citizens, and used rights-based provisions in the South African Constitution to secure poor people access to AIDS treatment. These legal challenges created the space for the articulation of a liberal democratic discourse on health citizenship. TAC's grassroots mobilisation and its legal challenges blurred the boundaries between the street and the courtroom. The Constitutional Court judges could not but be influenced by growing public support for TAC. The campaign achieved extraordinary media visibility and shaped public opinion through sophisticated networking and media imaging. It wase able to give passion and political and ethical content to the 'cold letter' of the Constitution and the 'cold facts' of AIDS statistics.

Flexible politics for flexible times

In December 2001, TAC's legal representatives successfully argued in the High Court of South Africa that the state had a constitutionally-bound obligation to promote access to health care, and that this could be extended to AIDS drug treatment.[22] This led to the government being ordered by the court to establish PMTCT programmes throughout the public health system. While the thrust of the TAC case focused on socio-economic rights, and specifically citizens' rights to health care, their lawyers raised broader issues relating to questions of scientific authority and expertise. The court was obliged to address the ongoing contestation over the scientific 'truth' on AIDS that raged between TAC, the trade unions, and health professionals on the one side, and government and the ANC on the other. By the end of 2003 it looked as if TAC and its allies had won this battle for ARV treatment.

Despite efforts to avoid being perceived as anti-government, TAC's criticism of President Mbeki's support for AIDS dissidents created dilemmas and difficulties. TAC activists were publicly accused by government spokespersons of being 'unpatriotic', 'anti-African' and salespersons of the international pharmaceutical industry. This locally situated cultural politics of race and national identity was addressed through a variety of strategies, including workshops, treatment literacy programmes and public meetings. TAC developed ways of combating what it perceived to be smear campaigns and attacks on its political credibility orchestrated by government spokespersons. It also managed the difficult feat of straddling the grey zones between cooperation with and opposition to government policies. Indeed, TAC's legal and political strategies reveal a clear understanding of the politics of contingency in contrast to an inflexible antagonistic politics of binaries: us and them.

TAC avoided being slotted into the conservative white camp through the creative reappropriation of locally embedded political symbols, songs and styles of the anti-apartheid struggle. For example, the Christopher Moraka Defiance Campaign resonated with the historic anti-*dompas* (pass law) defiance campaigns of the apartheid era. By mobilising township residents, especially working-class and unemployed black women, TAC challenged attempts by certain government officials to whitewash it as 'anti-black'. By bringing the trade union movement on board, TAC also challenged accusations that it was a front for white liberals, the drug companies, and other 'unpatriotic forces'. By positioning themselves as supporters of the ANC, SACP and COSATU Tripartite Alliance, TAC activists have

---

[22] The South African Constitution is unique in providing for water and housing (along with health care and a clean environment) as basic rights in the Bill of Rights.

managed to create a new space for critical engagement with the ANC government. They have also introduced new concepts of health citizenship that have raised questions about the relationship between science, medicine, rights and citizen participation in South Africa.

TAC's strategic engagement with politics of race and class emerged from the organisational memory of AIDS activists who participated in the United Democratic Front (UDF) in the 1980s. This expressed itself through songs at marches, demonstrations and funerals, and the regular press releases and conferences, website information dissemination, television documentaries and national and international networking. This political style is a sophisticated refashioning of 1980s modes of political activism, drawing on the courts, the media, and local and transnational advocacy networks, along with grassroots mobilisation and skilful negotiations with business and the state.

Perhaps the most important reason for the successes of TAC's grassroots mobilisation has been its capacity to provide poor and unemployed HIV-positive black South Africans with a biomedical and a psychological lifeline, often in contexts where they experience hostility and rejection from their communities, friends and families. The story of V (see above) draws attention to how experiences of sexual violence and AIDS can trump cultural nationalist ideologies and race solidarities. The politics of class, and the access to life-saving drugs for poor people, seemed to offer an alternative to an elite-driven politics of race and cultural identity.

Health activism in local spaces

In December 2003, TAC activist Lorna Mlofana, aged 21, was gang-raped at a Khayelitsha (Cape Town) shebeen toilet, and beaten to death when she told her attackers that she was HIV-positive. For a period after Mlofana's brutal murder many TAC activists in Khayelitsha were afraid to wear the TAC HIV Positive t-shirts. The Campaign's response to this traumatic event was to hold protests outside the Khayelitsha magistrate's court, and to launch educational 'blitzes' on trains and at clinics. Activists also made door-to-door visits to households in Town Two, the area in which Mlofana was killed, to educate people about AIDS. This shocking HIV/AIDS-related murder took place despite the fact that MSF and TAC had managed to establish exceptionally successful AIDS prevention and treatment programmes in Khayelitsha.

A number of studies have drawn attention to sexual violence and AIDS myths, conspiracies, stigma and denial in many parts of South Africa, showing how particularly pervasive they are in rural areas and poor communities that have had little exposure to AIDS activism, treatment literacy campaigns and grassroots mobilisation. It is also widely documented, for example, that in many parts of the country, women are not able to make independent decisions about contraception, or whether to take the HIV test and join ARV and PMTCT programmes if they are HIV-positive. These socio-cultural obstacles clearly have serious implications in terms of access to HIV programmes.

The parts of the country that have the highest rates of uptake for PMTCT and ARV programmes have tended to be the urban centres of the Western Cape, Kwa-

Zulu Natal (KZN) and Gauteng, areas where TAC and MSF activity has, until recently, tended to be concentrated.[23] NGO and social movement partnerships have played a significant role in creating the conditions for the uptake of bio-medical interventions such as PMTCT and ARV treatment. It would also seem that organisations are increasingly introducing new ideas about health citizenship in rural areas where traditional practices often clash with notions of female bodily autonomy and individual responsibility for one's health. In South Africa, a massive AIDS industry targeting an estimated 5.5 million South Africans living with AIDS is part of a global health intervention that involves the massive expansion of repro-ductive health, immunisation, and TB, malaria and AIDS programmes throughout the Global South. As will be discussed in the next chapter, these programmes are contributing towards establishing new forms of therapeutic citizenship (Nguyen 2005) that draw on liberal individualist conceptions of self-fashioning, 'responsi-bilised citizenship', and 'caring of the self' (Rose 2007).

Although TAC can be described as a rights-based social movement that uses the courts and constitutional rights to health care, it is also a grassroots, working-class social movement that goes beyond liberal individualism and rights talk. At the recent TAC national conference in Durban, I witnessed a particularly powerful session in which members gave impromptu testimony. Each highly charged tes-timony was followed by outbursts of song, dance and struggle chants: 'Long live, Zackie, long live. Long live, TAC, long live!' The following excerpts suggest that through grassroots mobilisation and treatment literacy campaigns TAC is able to articulate new forms of health/biological citizenship and political subjectivities that resonate amongst young, educated black youth in South African townships. Many of the testimonies demonstrated a sophisticated understanding of rights talk as well as intimate biomedical knowledge relating to AIDS treatment. They also expressed a quasi-religious sense of collective purpose, solidarity and belonging:

> I'm a person living with HIV. I received counselling before and after I tested. The counsellors at the hospital where I work as an admin clerk gave me nothing. I just found out I was HIV-positive and that was that. Three times I tried to commit suicide. Now I'm more positive than HIV-positive, thanks to TAC.
>
> (Thirty-something black man)

> When I go to my doctor I tell him exactly what medicines I need. He asks me if I've trained in medicine at the university. No, I say to him. It was TAC that taught me.
>
> (Thirty-something black woman)

> Thank you to MSF. My CD4 count was 28 now it is 543. Thank you to TAC.
>
> (Twenty-something black man)

> I'm Dudu. I was tested in 1996. In 1999 my CD4 count was below 200. I have lost many things in my life. But now with ARVs my CD4 count is 725 and the virus is undetected. I'm a person living with HIV. *Today I have a life. I can have a family. But it's painful when I take my medicine* [ARVs] *because I know someone is dying because he can't get treatment.*
>
> (Twenty-something black man, my emphasis)

---

[23] TAC and MSF have recently established treatment programmes in rural Lusikisiki (former Transkei) in the Eastern Cape Province.

These ritualised illness and treatment testimonies suggest that participants at the TAC conference in Durban had overcome stigma, fear, denial, witchcraft beliefs and other barriers to HIV/AIDS testing, disclosure and treatment. They also appear to have undertaken a quasi-religious conversion process that is discussed in more detail in the chapter that follows. This fervent belief in medical solutions expressed through public statements of positive living and commitment to ARV treatment, contrasts strikingly with the numerous obstacles to treatment access I encountered in 2003 during a visit to rural parts of Mpumalanga. While Nevirapine[24] was available at many of the PMTCT clinics, a dizzying array of socio-cultural obstacles, as well as political, logistical and capacity problems, seemed to stymie the implementation of PMTCT programmes at every turn.

Sociology professor Renee Fox, in a personal communication, January 2004, recounted to me her experiences in Khayelitsha during a discussion with a group of research fieldworkers from the area, who were preparing to conduct interviews on local attitudes to HIV/AIDS. Fox asked the fieldworkers whether it would be possible to avoid resistance to questions relating to witchcraft by framing the questions differently, for example, by asking whether the respondents thought that angry and envious thoughts and feelings, the breaking of certain taboos, or seeking the intervention of a magico-religious specialist to do harm to another, could cause AIDS. She was surprised by the responses:

> At first the group met what I said with total silence. But then they began to respond. One person said jokingly, 'There are those who believe that God will punish them [with AIDS] if they don't go to church on Sunday.' Another person suggested that others believed 'the ancestors' might punish you in this way if you broke taboos. Then, someone else exclaimed, 'How is it possible that in this beautiful, free land of ours' such an epidemic of AIDS could come to pass? This was a sheer outcry of a question of meaning. What followed rapidly were suggestions that some people believe that 'foreigners' can cause AIDS – 'foreigners' being defined as other black Africans immigrating to South Africa from surrounding countries, as well as whites; that condoms could cause AIDS (rather than prevent it); and that ARV treatment and modern Western medicine more generally could do harm. At the end of this discussion with this field team, I wasn't sure any longer whether they were simply describing beliefs of others, or whether they themselves subscribed to the same beliefs. (Renee Fox, personal communication)

Tobias Hecht, an anthropologist working in Mandela Park, Hout Bay, encountered similar views and was told by Xhosa-speaking residents that 'God sent AIDS to punish us for our sins', and that becoming HIV-positive through witchcraft was the most lethal mode of transmission (Tobias Hecht, personal communication, March 2004). Both Fox and Hecht are uncertain whether their informants shared these beliefs, or whether they were simply reporting on other members of the communities in which they lived. It is quite possible that people living in places such as Khayelitsha and Mandela Park, like most people, are able to believe in both universalist biomedical truth and spiritual/cultural interpretations of illness. The healing powers of western biomedicine, Christianity and the spiritual forces of the occult are not necessarily viewed as incompatible. These examples of double

---

24 Nevirapine is an anti-retroviral drug that is used both for the prevention of vertical transmission of HIV from mother to child as well as part of the triple-therapy ARV regimen.

or triple consciousness question public health arguments that it is necessary for patients to abandon traditional beliefs in order fully to embrace biomedical truth.

My initial impression from my visit to Mpumalanga was that, to improve access to AIDS treatment, rural villagers should be exposed to a strong dose of TAC and MSF health activism and grassroots mobilisation of the sort that emerged in the urban centres of Cape Town, Johannesburg and Durban. However, while there can be little doubt that TAC and MSF have contributed enormously towards creating the conditions conducive to the uptake of biomedical HIV/AIDS interventions such as ARV treatment, this does not mean that rank-and-file TAC members have been unambiguously converted to biomedicine. While many of the participants in the ARV trials at Khayelitsha appear to have accepted the biomedical truths and rights-based approaches to health citizenship promoted by their MSF doctors, this does not necessarily exclude beliefs in the occult or other faith-based and spiritual forms of healing. Conversion to mainstream AIDS science may be partial and precarious: for instance, a TAC activist recounted how even some of their seasoned volunteers had been seduced by President Mbeki's dissident views. Religious, spiritual and traditional explanations and modes of healing are significant contenders in the struggle to fight and make sense of HIV/AIDS. Again, Tobias Hecht and I visited the MSF clinic in Khayelitsha to find out what had happened to an HIV-positive TAC member who, we were told, had thrown her ARVs away after joining the local branch of the (Brazilian) Universal Church of the Kingdom of God (UCKG). An MSF nurse told us that TAC activists had successfully persuaded the woman to return to ARV treatment. We later visited a UCKG pastor who tried to convince us that numerous HIV-positive congregation members had become HIV-negative through prayer: 'If Jesus could heal leprosy, then why not AIDS?', he asked.

Despite the partial character of TAC and MSF's conversion process, it is nonetheless clear that they have contributed enormously towards combating AIDS fear and stigma, and promoting easier access to PMTCT and ARV treatment programmes. These forms of health activism also appear to have succeeded in overcoming many of the socio-cultural obstacles to HIV testing and treatment referred to above. They have contributed towards creating new forms of belonging, citizenship, scientific knowledge and subjectivity that resemble those emerging from the people's health movements in Europe as well as developing countries such as Brazil. Instead of being rejected by family, friends and community, many HIV-positive TAC members are now able to belong to local and global activist communities that recognise and celebrate their humanity and vitality; they are no longer the 'walking dead' to be pitied or avoided. They are 'more positive than HIV-positive, thanks to TAC'.[25] Politicising the right to health care has empowered citizens.

[25] Renee Fox, personal communication, reminded me that saying 'I am stronger now thanks to MSF and TAC' does not necessarily refer exclusively to physical health. It could also be a statement about the role of ARVs in producing a spiritual strength in the battle against the occult and 'evil' forces of envy and jealousy. This spiritual empowerment, however, does not mesh with TAC and MSF's stridently secular and scientific cosmology. As a result, public testimonies of the sort that were made at the TAC Durban Conference emphasised secular rationalist discourses on empowerment through access to scientific and medical knowledge.

However, there is a downside to this seeming wholesale endorsement of the power of biomedicine. In an interview with Eric Goemaere (Khayelitsha, 20 May 2004), an MSF doctor in Khayelitsha, it became clear that MSF and TAC are acutely aware of the Janus-like character of ARVs and other biomedical technologies. Goemaere pointed out that whereas anti-retroviral therapy can undoubtedly prolong lives, it can also become a conduit for the 'medicalisation of poverty' and the creation of dependencies on medical experts and drugs. Although MSF consciously seeks to counter disempowering and normalising biomedical discourses by stressing citizen rights to health care and medical and scientific knowledge, such messages are seldom heard in the public health clinics. Instead, clinic nurses and doctors tend to reproduce hierarchical and paternalistic expert–patient relations. Language, class, race, ethnic and education divides and socio-cultural barriers also collude to reproduce the passivity and disempowerment of working-class users of public health facilities.

The hierarchical and authoritarian cultures of many public health facilities can create obstacles in terms of access to AIDS programmes, particularly in areas untouched by social mobilisation and health activism. These problems are exacerbated in contexts where patriarchal ideas and practices prevent women from accessing health facilities, for instance, for HIV-testing and participation in PMTCT programmes. The testimonies of young women at the 2003 TAC conference (cited above) allude to TAC and MSF's challenges to deeply embedded patriarchal and biomedical ways of controlling female bodies and minds by creating the conditions for women to exercise agency in relation to male family members and medical experts.

While the dissident debate now appears to be mere history, stigma, fear, denial and patriarchal attitudes are likely to continue to be serious obstacles to AIDS prevention and treatment programmes. For example, 'Thembeka', a young HIV-positive AIDS counsellor in Mandela Park, Hout Bay, told me how she was struggling to access residents in this informal settlement. She mentioned that while her visits were appreciated when her HIV-positive 'clients' were seriously ill and desperately needed home-based care, they were furious with her when she visited them in *shebeens* and other public places, where, in the eyes of residents, her mere presence associated those she visited with AIDS.[26] They would 'disappear' when they were relatively healthy and reappear when they became critically ill. TAC, MSF, public health professionals and other civil society organisations clearly have their work cut out for them in places such as Mandela Park.

Health professionals, church groups, and organisations such as MSF and TAC are emerging as catalysts for attempts to democratise science and public health, often in contexts of chronic poverty, everyday violence, AIDS denial, and beliefs in witchcraft and other alternatives to AIDS science. It remains to be seen in what ways, if at all, these organisations and HIV/AIDS interventions are able to

---

[26] 'Thembeka' spoke of having tried, unsuccessfully, to use the AIDS counselling methods she learnt at Khayelitsha, where she receives ARV therapy at the MSF clinic. She reported that Mandela Park's HIV-positive residents remained in a state of AIDS denial, and that the two AIDS support groups in the area were clandestine as their members did not want to be exposed to the stigma so pervasive in the community.

challenge such socio-cultural obstacles. Nor is it clear to what degree they could unwittingly be promoting the dependencies and 'medicalisation of poverty' about which Goemaere expressed concern. It also remains to be seen how AIDS activists and public health professionals will address 'alternative' (non-biomedical) interpretations of disease and illness. Will a national ARV treatment programme extend normalising biomedical discourses and reduce citizens to docile consumers of medical technologies and scientific expertise? Or will citizens be able to engage with biomedicine in empowering ways?

Conclusion

South Africa's devastating HIV/AIDS statistics, President Mbeki's controversial support for the 'dissidents', and TAC's widely publicised court victories over both the South African government and the multinational pharmaceutical giants, thrust the South African AIDS pandemic onto the global stage. Mbeki's African nationalist response to the AIDS pandemic illustrates the workings of a cultural politics of identity that diverted attention from working-class and poor people's struggles for access to life-saving AIDS treatment that is accessible to the middle classes. The responses of African nationalists and dissidents within government and the ruling party clashed with the class and rights-based mobilisation of AIDS activists and trade unionists who insisted that ARVs be made freely available in public health facilities as part of citizens' constitutional rights to health care. The case study of these starkly contrasting responses to AIDS draws attention to the potential pitfalls as well as the emancipatory possibilities that exist for democratising science in a time of AIDS.

TAC's mode of activism captivated the imagination of AIDS activists, journalists and millions of supporters throughout the world: here was the archetypal David and Goliath epic. In their quest for AIDS drugs, a small group of committed activists were able to build a globally connected social movement – a form of practised citizenship – that successfully persuaded pharmaceutical giants and the South African government to put measures in place for the provision of AIDS treatment.

The AIDS pandemic, and the ways in which responses to it have unfolded in South Africa, raise important concerns about the social responsibilities of, and relationships between, the state, business and civil society. It has also drawn attention to the role of scientific expertise and trust in expert systems, as well as issues of political and scientific authority and moral legitimacy, and the ways in which publics relate to these. In addition to the profound confusion and uncertainty experienced by South African publics as a result of President Mbeki's questioning of conventional AIDS science, it has become apparent that people's interpretations of the AIDS pandemic are far more complex and differentiated than either the government or TAC originally anticipated. Journalists and researchers have uncovered a proliferation of AIDS myths and cultural interpretations of HIV/AIDS, including patriarchal conceptions of sexuality, which threaten to undermine treatment and prevention programmes. AIDS science and scientific authority were certainly undermined by the politicised nature of the dissident debate, but not all blame can be pinned onto the President.

TAC drew on a rights-based approach as well as grassroots mobilisation in working-class black communities. Its dramatic courtroom victories, along with its innovative forms of mobilisation, were part of a largely working-class struggle to gain access to life-saving drugs. It was also a campaign to assert the right of citizens to scientific knowledge, treatment information and the latest research findings: a post-apartheid expression of health citizenship.

TAC's mode of social mobilisation operated at a number of levels: global, national and local. At the global level, it challenged the intellectual property regime and drug pricing protocols and regulations imposed by the pharmaceutical industry; at the national level, it posed a fundamental challenge to the South African government's AIDS treatment policies; and at the local level, it mobilised working-class black communities, creating the conditions for the articulation of forms of health/biological citizenship as well as new gendered identities and subjectivities that challenged traditional and patriarchal ideas and practices. While TAC's mobilisation practices and treatment access campaigns operated at all three levels simultaneously, its activities have been, until recently, largely confined to urban areas, where it has drawn in young, black secondary-school leavers and students. It remains to be seen to what degree MSF and TAC will be able to extend their social mobilisation and treatment access campaigns to other contexts, for instance the countryside of the former homelands, where patriarchal cultures and the politics of shame and denial continue to frustrate efforts to make the public health system more accessible to HIV-positive people, especially women.[27] Is it possible to replicate and 'scale up' TAC and MSF's dramatic successes in urban centres such as Khayelitsha as part of the national ARV programme? What lessons from the MSF and TAC programmes in Khayelitsha and Lusikisiki can be exported to other ARV rollout sites?[28]

It also remains to be seen what role TAC/MSF will play in mediating these universalist biomedical understandings of disease and illness in South African communities where there are competing explanations for misfortune, ill-health, and sexuality. In what ways will MSF and TAC continue to be a catalyst for the spread of new notions of health citizenship, sexual rights and the democratisation of science in post-apartheid South Africa? The following chapter explores new forms of community-based AIDS activism that suggest ways of extending the reach of the successful rights-based approach of TAC.

[27] See S. Robins, 'Reclaiming Bodies, Extending Citizenship: Health Activism in a Time of AIDS' (unpublished paper, Association of Anthropology in Southern Africa conference, University of Cape Town, 24–7 August 2003).

[28] It is also unclear whether the South African government and public health officials responsible for running an extremely over-burdened public health system will agree, once and for all, to bury the 'dissident hatchet' and work together with TAC, MSF and other civil society organisations. While it is clear that many provincial and local government health managers and public health practitioners look favourably upon such partnerships, it is unclear whether the political fallout from the dissident debate will continue to stymie national government responses to the epidemic. In 2008 the prospects of state–civil society cooperation look reasonably optimistic, notwithstanding the health minister's bizarre attempts to promote garlic, beetroot and olive oil as part of her anti-AIDS nutrition cocktail.

6

Rights Passages from 'Near Death' to 'New Life'
AIDS Activism & New HIV-identities
in South Africa

Introduction[1]

This chapter investigates how the moral politics of AIDS activism in South Africa is contributing towards new forms of subjectivity, identity and citizenship. Whereas Chapter 5 focused on the politics of AIDS and the emergence of a rights-based social movement, this chapter is concerned with the relationship between individual and collective experiences and interpretations of the extreme experiences of the illness and stigmatisation of AIDS sufferers. I argue that it is precisely the extremity of 'near death' experiences of full-blown AIDS, and the profound stigma and 'social death' associated with the later stages of the disease, that produce the conditions for AIDS survivors' commitment to forms of 'responsibilised citizenship' (Rose 2007) and social activism. It will be argued that it is the NGO and social movement involvement in the mediation and retelling of these traumatic experiences that can contribute towards facilitating the individual's commitment to 'responsible' lifestyles and 'positive living'. It is the profound negativity of stigma and social death that animates the activist's construction of a new positive HIV-positive identity and understanding of what it means to belong to a social movement and community of people living with AIDS.

This case study, like the others in this book, highlights the ambiguous and contradictory character of rights-based approaches to political mobilisation in post-apartheid South Africa. For instance, it questions widely held assumptions about the individualising and depoliticising nature of rights talk and biomedical

[1] This chapter could not have been written without the generous assistance of numerous people including Phumzile Nywagi, Akhona Ntsaluba, Chris Colvin, Andrew Boulle, Jean Comaroff, Lauren Müller, Ruth Cornick, Herman Reuter, Kees van der Waal and numerous other TAC and MSF activists. I would also like to thank John Gaventa, Melissa Leach, Ian Scoones, Bettina von Lieres, and other participants in the joint School of Government, University of the Western Cape, and Institute for Development Studies, Sussex University project on Citizenship, Participation and Accountability. I am particularly indebted to Brahm Fleisch for his suggestion that I turn to Victor Turner's analysis of ritual processes. I am also especially grateful to Melissa Leach and Chris Colvin for exceptionally helpful comments on earlier versions of this paper.

discourses on 'responsibilised' citizenship (Barry, Osborne and Rose 1996; Rose, 2007). Rather than viewing public health conceptions of 'responsibilisation' as mere reflections of the cultural hegemony of biocapital (Sundar Rajan 2006) and the downsizing neoliberal state's imperatives of governance-at-a-distance, this case study draws attention to the diverse political rationalities and identities that emerge at the interface of biomedicine, the individual patient-citizen and NGO-social movement activism. The outcomes of these complex interactions include hybrid political discourses that defy the enduring binary categories of citizens and subjects, liberal and communitarian and so on. The illness narratives and treatment testimonies discussed in this case draw attention to the improvisational and situational character of responses to AIDS activist interventions and public health programmes in post-apartheid South Africa.

The case explores how the combination of illness experiences and enrolment in the Treatment Action Campaign (TAC) and *Médecins Sans Frontières* (MSF) treatment programmes has, in many cases, dramatically altered the lives, subjectivities, identities, life-narratives and futures of people living with HIV/AIDS (PLWHAs). It investigates these issues in the context of AIDS activist struggles for free treatment in South Africa's public health sector. While these activist organisations are generally understood as rights-based social movements (Friedman and Mottiar 2004), the illness narratives and treatment testimonies that are analysed in this chapter suggest that experiences of illness, treatment and participation in TAC and MSF can produce radical transformations in subjectivity and identity that go well beyond conventional liberal democratic conceptions of 'rights' and citizenship. At the same time, these changes in subjectivity can, in certain cases, produce the kinds of responsibilised citizens that public health professionals believe are required for safe and effective AIDS treatment to take place.

There has been considerable public debate in the South African media about the need to balance individual rights and responsibilities when it comes to HIV/AIDS. This is not surprising given the widespread fear that poor treatment adherence could produce multi-drug resistant HIV. Some public health professionals have sought to justify compulsory testing and status notification, and the overriding of individual rights to treatment for those who show signs that they may not be able to adhere to treatment (*Cape Times*, 15 April 2005). For example, Professor Solly Benatar, the director of the Bioethics Centre at the University of Cape Town, has called for a balance between the rights of individuals and the public health needs of society. To maximise adherence to ARV treatment, he argued, required that patients take some responsibility for their own health (ibid.). There have also been calls from progressive public health circles for a new contract between provider and client that would replace the paternalistic surveillance model of direct observation therapy (DOT) TB treatment. The latter, it is argued, cannot work with life-long ARV treatment, and what is needed are responsibilised citizens and knowledgeable and empowered HIV-positive clients. But how can these new rights and responsibilities approaches take hold in contexts characterised by extreme forms of AIDS stigma, shame, denial and fear? What role should the state, public health practitioners and civil society organisations play in prompting responsibility in such contexts? What kinds of subjectivities, and social, economic and cultural conditions, are necessary for safe and effective treatment of HIV/AIDS?

Drawing on illness narratives and treatment testimonies, I will argue that these rights and responsibilities approaches to public health, important as they are, do not adequately acknowledge the consequences of the profoundly traumatic and transformative nature of HIV illness and treatment experiences. Neither do they take sufficient cognisance of the complex mix of religious, communal, biomedical and activist mediations and narrations of illness and treatment experiences, and how these can, under certain conditions, contribute towards creating the kinds of responsibilised citizens that public health practitioners and rights activists desire. Liberal individualist rights talk, I argue, does not address the radically transformative character of the new biosocial subjectivities and HIV-positive identities that I discuss in this chapter. The latter are not simply the product of liberal modernist discourses on the rights-bearing citizen. Instead, they are forged in the course of the traumatic journeys from 'near death' ('bare life') to 'new life' that I refer to as rights passages.

The central character in this case is Phumzile Nywagi, a forty-five-year-old activist living with AIDS in Cape Town. In Chapter 7 I discuss how Phumzile, a former MSF and TAC activist, founded Khululeka, a support group for HIV-positive men. Khululeka is an offshoot from the Treatment Action Campaign (TAC) and was formed largely in response to Phumzile's belief that township men were sexually and socially 'irresponsible' and were conspicuously absent from public clinics and HIV/ AIDS support groups. Whereas TAC is a rights-based movement largely consisting of women, Phumzile and his support group have attempted to address specifically men's issues, including dominant male sexual cultures. This chapter focuses on how activists such as Phumzile have imbibed MSF and TAC's commitment to AIDS activism and liberal democratic conceptions of rights and responsibilities.

The case shows how a new moral politics is being constructed by AIDS activists and people living with AIDS through the deployment of religious, communal, biomedical, rights-based and social activist discursive framings. People living with AIDS often draw on these multiple framings to make sense of their illness and social suffering. These framings, I argue, can contribute to the production of 'positive' HIV-positive identities and new forms of sociality and citizenship for AIDS sufferers in Third World settings where stigma and social isolation are pervasive and access to treatment continues to be a life-and-death struggle. It will be argued that while these framings may draw on rights-based discourses, they exceed liberal individualist conceptions of citizenship in their engagement with religious, communal, social and existential dimensions of illness and suffering.

Animating AIDS activism: from 'bare life' to 'new life'

Hannah Arendt (1958) noted that the modern state had become increasingly concerned with biological existence and the management of 'life processes'. Similarly,

Giorgio Agamben (1998) claims that both modern and archaic political orders have been preoccupied with the capacity to control life by excluding it from meaningful social and political existence. Drawing on the ideas of both Arendt and Agamben, Jean Comaroff argues that in the modern world the management and politics of 'bare life' has shifted centre-stage: it is both the object of state enforcement and the subject of projects of democratic emancipation and citizenship (Comaroff n.d.: 14). According to Comaroff, the political history of the West leads us to a situation whereby there is 'an unprecedented capacity and concern to enhance life [which] is rivalled only by the power to destroy it' (ibid.). Comaroff reminds us that Agamben draws on *homo sacer* – the archaic Roman law figure who 'could be killed but not sacrificed' – to illustrate that modern life is 'simultaneously sacred, and utterly dispensable' (ibid.: 15). Whereas Agamben is specifically concerned with the relation between *homo sacer* and sovereign power, Comaroff notes that scholars such as Joao Biehl (2001) and Ulrike Kistner (2004) are beginning to draw connections between this Roman law figure and 'the Third World HIV/AIDS sufferer: a being condemned to callous exclusion, to death without meaning or sacrificial value, in an age of widespread humanitarian empathy; a being left untreated in an era of pharmacological salvation' (Comaroff n.d.:15). Comaroff draws our attention to a moral politics of AIDS activism in places like Brazil and South Africa that insists on 'making death sacrificial once more'. In other words, through NGO and social movement activism death is made socially meaningful.

Pain, illness and suffering are often represented as inherently private and physical phenomena that have little to do with the social world. Yet, numerous scholars have pointed out that the experience of pain and suffering is fundamentally social. For anthropologists this observation is neither new nor surprising. Writing in the 1960s, Victor Turner (1961, 1969) showed how Ndembu interpreted the sick individual body as a sign of disease and disorder in the wider social body; here, healing involved the realignment of the social order. Biomedicine, by contrast, tends to depoliticise and individualise illness. Paul Farmer is amongst a number of scholars who have challenged these depoliticising and individualising discourses by drawing attention to broader social, political and economic structures that determine the epidemiological distribution and subjective experience of disease and suffering in the Third World. Farmer (2004) draws on the concept of 'structural violence' to show how conditions of chronic poverty, gender inequality, traumatic violence, and infectious diseases limit the life choices of the women he encounters at his HIV/AIDS clinic in rural Haiti. These patients are the literal embodiment of global structures of inequality.

Farmer's linking of the individual AIDS body to structural processes resembles anthropological accounts of how small-scale societies interpret the sick individual body as a sign of disease within the broader social body. South African AIDS activists belonging to TAC and MSF make similar connections between individual PLWHAs and the body politic. Here the wider social world is characterised by conditions of unequal and inadequate health care reproduced by the greed and profiteering of global pharmaceutical companies. These health inequalities are also understood by activists as the product of a legacy of apartheid racism, as well as more recent forms of state indifference and inaction in relation to the provision of AIDS treatment in the public sector. With the South African government's decision in October 2003 to establish a national ARV programme, activist attention has increasingly shifted towards monitoring this programme and drawing attention to the regional inequalities and 'blockages' within the national public health system.

South Africa now has one of the largest AIDS treatment programmes in the world. In 2008 only 371,731 (42%) of an estimated 889,000 people who needed anti-retroviral therapy were accessing free treatment through the public health system. This limited access to treatment is particularly worrying given current estimates that there are between five and six million HIV-positive South Africans. Notwithstanding the introduction of a massive national ARV programme, AIDS activists find themselves having to continue to challenge the global pharmaceutical industry's patents, policies and pricing structures, the national leadership's perceived lack of political will when it comes to treatment, as well as AIDS dissidents who persist in questioning the link between HIV and AIDS, the scale of the AIDS pandemic and the efficacy and safety of antiretroviral therapy. This chapter, however, is concerned with another dimension of TAC activism, namely its capacity to create the conditions for the production of new subjectivities and identities out of the traumatic experiences of illness and stigmatisation of individual AIDS sufferers. The study focuses on the ways in which experiences of illness, treatment and activism can together contribute towards profound changes in the lives of people with HIV/AIDS.

Revisiting 'the ritual process': treatment activism and 'responsibilised citizens'

One useful way of interpreting these profound transformations is Victor Turner's pioneering work on the ritual process. Turner's analysis provides a rich heuristic device and analytical lens through which to interpret how the extremity of 'near death' experiences of full-blown AIDS, followed by 'miraculous' recovery through ARV treatment, can produce the conditions for AIDS survivors' commitment to 'new life' and social activism. It is the activist mediation and the retelling of these traumatic experiences, I will argue, that facilitates TAC's highly successful grassroots mobilisations. It will also be argued that it is precisely these processes of illness, stigma and treatment that provide activists with the raw materials with which to construct rights-based politics and new HIV-positive identities and social solidarities. Rights-based mobilisation, it is argued, is often the outcome of these kinds of transformative experiences.

These activist mediations of illness and treatment experiences can be distinguished from AIDS treatment in the public sector, which is shaped by the conventional doctor–patient dyad and highly technicist and depoliticised modes of biomedical intervention in the private spaces of doctors' consultancy rooms. By contrast, TAC activism creates the conditions for more collectivist responses to HIV and treatment. This AIDS activist culture has been very present at the two MSF-Department of Health ARV programmes in Khayelitisha, Cape Town, and Lusikisiki, Eastern Cape Province. Whereas public health practitioners report that most of their HIV/AIDS patients wish to retain anonymity and invisibility at all costs, TAC successfully advocates the transformation of the stigma of AIDS into a badge of pride that is publicly displayed on T-shirts at township funerals, demonstrations, workshops and other public spaces. It is through these activist mediations that it becomes possible for the social reintegration and revitalisation of large numbers of isolated and stigmatised AIDS sufferers into a social movement and a caring community. However, the majority of public sector ARV programmes in South Africa are characterised by hierarchical and authoritarian doctor–nurse–patient interactions. Doctors and nursing staff working in these settings also believed that most of their HIV-positive patients would probably want to avoid involvement in AIDS activism precisely because of its emphasis on public visibility and disclosure (Dr Ruth Cornick, personal commitment). So what kinds of social and ritual processes can create the conditions for people living with AIDS to turn AIDS stigma, isolation and shame into a 'badge of pride'?

In *The Recovering Alcoholic*, Norman Denzin (1987: 12) draws attention to the role of Alcoholics Anonymous (AA) treatment rituals in 'the transformations in experience that produce situational and long-term commitments to the identity of the "recovering alcoholic"'. Denzin describes these AA rituals as processes of 'adult socialisation' and 'identity transformation or conversion', terms that 'refer to the process by which the self of the person actively enters into the acquisition of new self-images, new languages of self, new relations with others, and new bonds or ties to the social order' (ibid.: 19). In his account of 'the social worlds' of the recovering alcoholic, Denzin identifies the central role of AA rituals – the 'Twelve Steps' and 'Twelve Traditions' and rituals of storytelling – in the treatment and recovery process (ibid.: 118-21). While ritual may not appear at first glance to be a useful and appropriate concept for describing AIDS activism and social mobilisation, this chapter will draw on Turner's (1969) analysis of the ritual process to understand the extraordinary biosocial power of ARV treatment and AIDS activism in a context of hyper-stigma and AIDS traumas of social and biological death. This will be done by analysing the treatment narratives of two AIDS activists on life-long ARV treatment. Discussion of these case studies will rely on Turner's use of Arnold Van Gennep's (1960) identification of the three stages of rites of passage: separation; liminality/communitas; and reintegration. Ritual analysis offers analytical insights into the radical transformational power of these death-to-life transitions that PWAs personally experience, or witness. Turner's work can also throw light on the social status shifts that take place when the stigmatised and isolated sick recover and become reintegrated into TAC as healthy and socially active members of society.

While it is problematic to generalise beyond these individual cases, I suggest that the two illness and treatment testimonies analysed below do indeed resonate with narratives of AIDS experience that are widely shared and circulated within TAC. These narratives have become part of the collective cultural repertoire of

TAC even though not all members have personally been through these illness and treatment experiences. Although AIDS activists may not frame illness and treatment experiences through ritual analysis, it would seem that the transformations and transitions from 'near death' to 'new life' can be illuminated through the analytical heuristic of rights of passage. But what is the nature of these transformations and how do we relate these to questions of citizenship and subjectivity?

AIDS activism in South Africa shares similarities with identity-based illness movements elsewhere in the world (Epstein 1996; Petryna 2002). Concepts such as 'biological citizenship' (Petryna ibid.)[2] speak to a range of illness-based movements that have mobilised around nuclear radiation, breast cancer, psychiatric illnesses and HIV/AIDS. As was mentioned earlier, 'lay expertification' (Epstein ibid.) and 'citizen science' (Irwin 1995) are increasingly used to describe citizen responses to unpredictable and poorly managed health and environmental hazards. These developments, which often result in citizen scepticism and distrust of mainstream science and expertise, are linked to what Ulrich Beck (1992) and Anthony Giddens (1991) refer to as contemporary conditions of reflexive modernity and 'world risk society'. For Beck and Giddens, both of whom are writing specifically about the advanced capitalist countries of the West, citizens have become increasingly distrustful of scientists and the scientific findings produced by governments and business. It is within this context that 'citizen science' (Irwin 1995), 'expertification from below' and the making of biological citizens is taking place. These processes intersect with the popular fascination – at least in the US and Europe – with 'risk factor' epidemiology, a technicist discourse that involves ever finer calibration and endless attempts to control risk in every aspect of our lives (Dr Chris Colvin, personal correspondence).

TAC and MSF activists argue that they are not only interested in medical treatment, but that they are also concerned with creating empowered citizens who understand the connections between biomedicine and the wider social world and political economy of health. This is evident in their legal challenge to the drug patents and pricing structures of the global pharmaceutical companies (see Chapter 5). TAC activists also share similar concerns with the Northern illness-based movements that have emerged as a result of citizen perceptions of inadequate scientific and government responses to a range of health and environmental hazards, for example, BSE, foot and mouth, biotechnology and GMOs, pesticides, AIDS, global warming and so on. TAC also has its roots in distrust of government's response to the pandemic, especially President Mbeki's flirtation with AIDS dissident science

---

[2] Adriana Petryna (2002) has written about how, following the Chernobyl disaster, the newly independent Ukrainian state, radiation research clinics and NGOs 'mediated an informal economy of illness and claims to what I refer to as "biological citizenship" – a massive demand for but selective access to a form of social welfare based on scientific and legal criteria that both acknowledge injury and compensate for it.' Such struggles for biological citizenship unfolded in a context of the failure of the Ukrainian state to address massive unemployment, hyper-inflation and pervasive corruption. Within this context sufferers became dependent on being able to make 'claims for biomedical resources, social equity, and human rights' (Petryna, 2002: 192). Similar processes have been observed in relation to struggles by unemployed and poverty-stricken South African citizens for access to disability grants provided by the post-apartheid state to HIV-positive people with CD4 counts below 200.

and his government's initial reluctance to provide antiretroviral treatment to AIDS sufferers. It is this broad range of health and environmental concerns that are driving the growth of these illness–based social movements.

While the linking of biology and health to identity and social movements is certainly not new, what are new are the ways in which biological identities, and the interest groups formed in their name, are emerging in different parts of the world (Petryna 2002: 14). These movements have important implications in terms of extending liberal democratic notions of citizenship. In South Africa, for example, there has been a recent call for public health experts for a new contract between provider and client (see Coetzee and Schneider 2004). The advocates of this contract suggest that the passive and paternalistic surveillance model of direct observation therapy (DOT) TB treatment is not a viable solution for life-long ARV treatment. Instead what is needed, they argue, are highly motivated, 'responsibilised' and knowledgeable HIV-positive clients. But they do not seem to be able to provide clear indications as to how the public health system will be able to make this seismic shift from DOT paternalism to a more client-centred approach to HIV/AIDS.

It is perhaps not entirely coincidental that 'responsibilisation' also appears in the recent work of political theorists writing about contemporary liberal rationalities of government (see Barry *et al.* 1996). Here the term refers to the ways in which, under liberalism and neo-liberalism, 'the governed are encouraged, freely and rationally, to conduct themselves' (ibid.: 29). Barry, Osborne and Rose argue that neo-liberal rationalities of government encourage the governed to become responsible for issues previously held to be the responsibility of government authorities (ibid.). These ideas about responsibilised citizens are clearly by-products of this post-socialist and (neo)liberal age. But how do people living with AIDS engage with these calls for a new contract between health providers and empowered and responsibilised clients?

'AIDS is in my blood': Illness narratives and treatment testimonies

'AIDS has been a "blessing in disguise"'
'Thembeka' (not her actual name) is a thirty-something HIV-positive TAC activist in Lusikisiki, a small rural town in the former Transkei homeland in the Eastern Cape. She told me that discovering her HIV status and joining TAC and the MSF ARV treatment programme had dramatically improved her life: 'Thanks to TAC and MSF I'm flying. I've got wings to fly.' I recall being shocked when Thembeka first described her experience of HIV as a 'blessing in disguise'. Yet, as I got to know her, it became clear that being tested for HIV, joining TAC and the MSF ARV programme in Lusikisiki had indeed ushered in for her a new and better life. She recalled the trauma of sexual abuse by an uncle as a young girl, being sent away to stay with her mother's friends as a teenager while her younger sister stayed at home and attended a good 'Model C' school. She also tearfully recollected a violent gang rape by four youths and being unable to tell her parents about it because she feared that they would not believe her. Her rape led to pregnancy and her decision

to have an abortion, while her later discovery of her HIV status led to her decision to have a sterilisation operation.

> After I had my VCT [Voluntary Counselling & Testing] the counsellor told me that I'm HIV positive and that all my dreams are finished and I'm going to just die. And then they told me that all my kids would be HIV-positive. It's either I'll condomise, or if my husband sometimes doesn't want to use condoms then I should just use sterilisation. That's the way that they can help me. Because the more babies I have the more quickly I will die.

Thembeka's life story included accounts of child sexual abuse, rape, abortion, sterilisation and the onset of serious debilitating illness, culminating in her discovery in 2001 that both she and her baby were HIV-positive: 'I was very sick but then I found TAC and MSF and my life changed ... *TAC is my mother, MSF is my father*'. While her mother, who was a nurse, subscribed to the Minister of Health's controversial nutritional diet of garlic, lemons, olive oil and the 'African potato' for HIV-positive people, Thembeka's involvement with MSF and TAC led to her rejection of these alternative and traditional remedies and her participation in antiretroviral therapy at the MSF programme in Lusikisiki. The health minister's promotion of this nutritional advice was interpreted by AIDS activists such as Thembeka as tacit support for the dissidents' claims that ARVs were dangerously toxic. As her health improved under ARV treatment, Thembeka became integrated into the closely-knit and supportive network of TAC activists and MSF doctors and nurses. She learnt AIDS awareness training skills and acquired basic scientific knowledge about HIV/AIDS, prevention and treatment. She was also personally handed her ARVs by former president Nelson Mandela when he officially launched the ARV programme in Lusikisiki in 2003. When I met her in 2004 she was being headhunted by NGOs in the Eastern Cape but had decided to stay on as an MSF treatment literacy practitioner (TLP) and youth organiser in Lusikisiki. She spoke about her work as 'preaching the gospel'.

'I am like a Born Again, ARVs are now my life'

Phumzile,[3] the founder of Khululeka (see Chapter 7), told me how in 2001 he became desperately ill. He had headaches, dizziness, he suffered from a range of other opportunistic infections, he had lost almost 30 kilograms, his CD4 count[4] was down to 110, his viral load was 710,000, he could not walk, he was barely conscious at times, and he secluded himself in a room in his sister's house waiting for death. On 12 November 2001 he became one of the first 50 clients to participate in MSF's ARV treatment programme in Khayelitsha. His recovery was dramatic: after six months his viral load had dropped to 215,000, his CD4 went up and he was feeling much stronger. When I met Phumzile in 2004, his viral load was unde-

---

[3] Taped interviews with Phumzile Nywagi were conducted in Cape Town on 15 September and 4 October 2005. I also engaged with Phumzile over a number of years and thank him for his friendship, insights, courage and generosity.

[4] The CD4 count refers to the number of CD4 cells (T-helper lymphocytes with the CD4 cell surface marker). CD4 counts are used for a variety of purposes, including to assess a person's immune status, susceptibility to opportunistic infections, the need for Antiretroviral Therapy (ART) and opportunistic Infections (OI) prophylaxis and for defining AIDS. In South Africa a CD4 count of less than 200 is an indicator that a person needs to begin ART. It is also used to define when a person living with HIV is able to access the Disability Grant.

tectable and his CD4 count was 584. He had also become something of an AIDS celebrity and was regularly interviewed by journalists, filmmakers and academics about his experiences – for instance, he had represented South Africa at a Southern African Development Community (SADC) meeting in Lesotho on AIDS, and he was in demand from medical and social science researchers involved in HIV/AIDS research projects.

At the time of writing this chapter, Phumzile was working at a private health insurance company where he tele-counselled HIV-positive clients who were referred to the call centre by general practitioners who detected treatment adherence and related problems. As a result of requests from some clients for face-to-face meetings, Phumzile sometimes visited them at their homes. Even though the call centre was established to create the conditions of anonymity and confidentiality, Phumzile's own seropositive status and his highly personal style of tele-counselling elicited requests for more personal forms of interaction. As a result he spent many weekends visiting people living with AIDS in Cape Town and elsewhere in the country. As he put it: 'I am committed to my AIDS work. *AIDS is in my blood.*' Tele-counselling could not adequately meet his own needs for more personal face-to-face interactions.

Clinical indicators such as 'normal' CD4 counts and 'undetectable viral loads' do not adequately convey the sense of social, psychological and spiritual recovery that Phumzile and others have experienced on their journeys from 'near death' to 'new life'. Neither do these indicators account for why Phumzile, like Thembeka, viewed HIV as 'a blessing in disguise'. For Phumzile, getting his life back through ARV treatment was a gift from God that he could not afford to squander:

> I'm not a church-goer. My faith comes from the time I got sick … In the bible there is the story of a sick beggar on the road. Jesus comes by and tells the beggar to stand up. And he stands up. The miracle of Jesus revived him from death so that he could heal other people through the belief that Jesus is on earth. Faith is in yourself. If you don't believe in yourself, who do you believe in? God brought me back to life for a purpose. He wants me to go out there and talk to people. He's giving me another chance. A day could cost me a lot if I don't speak about HIV … At Groote Schuur [Hospital] I prayed a lot. I was thinking of my children growing up without their father's love, support and guidance … *I am like a born again. ARVs, that's where my commitment comes from. It's like committing yourself to life because the drugs are a life time thing. ARVs are now my life.*

At the 2003 TAC national conference in Durban, I witnessed a particularly powerful session in which members gave impromptu testimony of their treatment experiences. Each highly charged testimony was followed by outbursts of song, dance and struggle chants: 'Long live, Zackie, long live. Long live, TAC, long live!' (see Chapter 5). As was mentioned in the previous chapter, these treatment testimonies – with their references to CD4 counts, viral loads and the role of TAC in giving 'new life' – seem to blur the lines between science and religion, medicine and spirituality, and technology and magic. Even though TAC is a modernist and secular organisation, the quasi-religious quality of these testimonies was evident in Phumzile's testimony at the Durban meeting in 2003. The testimony also expresses the sense of personal empowerment that comes from having survived the passage from 'near death' to recovery:

> I'm Phumzile from Cape Town in the Western Cape. I was diagnosed in 2001 three days after my birthday. I was very sick. When you get sick you just ignore it. You say, 'Oh, it's just the flu'. You're in the denial stage. You say your neighbour is a witch … We thought this disease belonged to other people elsewhere in Africa. From my point of view HIV is real, it's here. *I never thought I would be here today. I couldn't stand, I was sick. My CD4 count was 110 and my viral load was 710,000. Then I started ARVs with MSF in Khayelitsha. Now I'm strong.*

Phumzile's double-entendre, 'AIDS is in my blood', captures the extraordinary agency and sense of purpose that Phumzile and many other activists living with AIDS seem to share.

Discussion of the treatment testimonies: the ritual process revisited

Turner's method of ritual analysis offers a valuable way to interpret the processes of personal transformation in the context of social movements. In *The Ritual Process* (1969), Turner identifies three stages of 'rites de passage' – separation, liminality/communitas and reintegration. It would seem possible, based on the treatment narratives discussed earlier, that the extremity of the forms of stigma, ostracisation and isolation that PWAs experience are analogous to the stage of ritualised 'separation' identified by Turner (see Biehl 2005). During this first stage the individual becomes sick, is afflicted with opportunistic infections and may already be in an advanced stage of AIDS. The illness may be understood by sick persons, family members and neighbours to be the work of *abathakathi* (witch-craft), a sign of having been chosen by the ancestors to be a *sangoma* (diviner), or simply an 'ordinary' illness such as flu or tuberculosis. Alternatively, the onset of these illnesses may lead to testing and the confirmation of an HIV-positive status. This extreme state of illness often results in the withdrawal of the sick person from everyday social spaces. The 'smell of death' may also heighten stigmatisation, ritualised avoidance and social and physical isolation by neighbours and family members. For example, 'Nomsa', a twenty-year-old HIV-positive woman I met in Lusikisiki in the Eastern Cape Province, spoke of how, upon disclosing her HIV-positive status to her family, she was given her own plates and utensils to eat with. Thereafter her stepfather chased her from his home and she moved to her mother's home. Isolation is also produced by the illness itself. An HIV clinician who works at an ARV rollout site in Cape Town tried to explain to me the obstacles to com-municating with patients with fully blown AIDS. 'They are so sick that it is often very difficult to have a conversation with them. They are sometimes like walking skeletons.' These descriptions are strikingly similar to the *musselmans* ('the walk-ing dead') of the concentration camps that Primo Levi (1979) wrote about in 'The Drowned and the Saved'.

In the second phase the sick person may seek biomedical treatment for oppor-tunistic infections, join a TAC support group, and enrol, depending on clinical indicators, for ARV treatment with MSF. The patient-activist learns basic scientific and biomedical knowledge about HIV/AIDS, including its symptoms and ARV treatment. During this stage patients are in a state of liminality as their future health status remains precarious and uncertain. They are betwixt and between in that it is not clear whether they are dying or on the path to recovery and health. They may have to wait to find out whether the drugs will work and whether there will be serious side-effects. Meanwhile, recruitment into TAC allows them access to a supportive community and non-hierarchical social space that is analogous to the experience of 'communitas' that Turner describes as characterising states of liminality.

Finally, the recovery of the patient-activist with HIV/AIDS can be likened to Turner's third phase of 'reincorporation'. In this third stage, the individual starts getting physically and psychologically well, the CD4 count increases, the viral load drops, and the person begins putting on weight and rediscovers his or her appetite for food, sex and sociality. This phase usually involves social incorporation into the TAC and and possibly also the wider community and society. It can transform the stigmatised and dying AIDS sufferer into an activist-citizen empowered with knowledge about HIV/AIDS and an ability to speak out in public spaces. Of course there is no inexorable linear treatment trajectory, and rejection and expulsion from community cannot be excluded as a possible treatment outcome. For Phumzile and Thembeka, however, this phase culminated in personal empowerment and spiritual awakening that convinced them 'HIV is a blessing in disguise'. TAC members with HIV/AIDS are hereby reinstated into the social world as human beings with dignity; they have a new positive HIV-positive status. In the case of Phumzile and Thembeka it was clear this process of social reintegration also involved a commitment to a 'new life' and social activism. This is what I mean by the biosocial passage from 'near death' to 'new life.'

While it is clearly not useful to force too tight a fit between Turner's model of the ritual process and the actual experiences and subjectivities of patient-activists with HIV/AIDS, this approach helps to account for why ARV treatment and TAC mobilisation appears to have been so successful at reconfiguring the stigma, isolation and suffering of AIDS into a positive and life-affirming HIV-positive identity and quasi-religious commitment to 'new life' and social activism. In this sense it extends social movement theories beyond those that simply attribute activist commitments to instrumental rationality, rational choice, education and conscientisation.

Turner's *The Ritual Process* is also instructive in its identification of common themes and structural features in millenarian religious movements, hippies and Franciscans; all these movements comprise marginal, or self-marginalised, people who are committed to the eradication of distinctions based on inequality and property. They are dedicated to the levelling of status and a communitarian ethos of unselfish commitment to collectively shared ideals. According to Turner, these movements strive to instantiate a permanent state of liminality and communitas – a statusless egalitarianism – that is not that different to the middle passage of 'traditional' rites of passage.

Like the social groups identified by Turner – millenarians, hippies and Franciscans – TAC consists largely of 'social marginals' – that is the sick and stigmatised poor, especially young unemployed black women. It is not surprising that this social category of 'marginals' would be drawn to a social movement that strives to eradicate distinctions based on status and hierarchy. These women are either HIV positive themselves or they have family members who have been deeply affected by the epidemic. They are also in many instances members of a generation that the liberation struggle has left behind. Unlike the high profile anti-apartheid activists of the 1980s, the majority of whom are now in government or business, TAC's rank-and-file members are generally without jobs and career prospects. This post-revolutionary generation of young people are caught in liminal space – betwixt and between structural marginalisation and the dream of post-apartheid liberation. Many of them do not have the material means, education or cultural capital to move beyond this structural location of marginality and liminality. In addition, they face the very real threat of social and biological death from AIDS, making it unlikely that they will be able to move through the life cycle rituals and trajectories of personhood of their parents' generation. Whereas Turner's social movements embraced liminality as a positive space, it would seem that TAC consists of reluctant members of a marginalised social category trapped in the zone of liminality in which the transition from youth to adulthood and elder status is being blocked by structural unemployment and the lethal equation: sex=death. Such circumstances make it extremely difficult to participate in social and biological reproduction and life cycle rituals. It is here, in the shadow of social and biological death, that the combination of ARVs and TAC offers such a compelling possibility for 'new life'.

The limits of social movement theories

Scholars working within science and technology studies (STS) have extended the scope of the social movements literature by addressing new forms of citizen participation and social mobilisation in the fields of biotechnology, biomedicine, environmental activism and so on (Epstein 1996; Leach *et al.* 2005, Rose 2007). This new direction in science studies also intersects with a growing literature that focuses on the diverse ways in which biomedical technologies are radically constituting new subjectivities and forms of citizenship (see Petryna 2002; Biehl, 2001, 2004, 2005; Nguyen, 2005;[5] Rose 2007). This case study has focused specifically on the ways in which treatment activism and the introduction of antiretroviral therapy (ART) within the public health system have transformed subjectivities

[5] Vinh-Kim Nguyen (2005: 126) uses the concept of *therapeutic citizenship* to describe everyday practices and techniques that produce new kinds of subjects and forms of life – AIDS activists, resistant viruses, and therapeutic citizens. For example, Nguyen writes about African AIDS activists who use their activist networks to get invited to European AIDS conferences so that they can access ARVs; in many cases they remain in Europe in order to stay on treatment. For these activists access to treatment depends upon developing social relations and capitalising on social networks (2005: 133). Nguyen's notions of therapeutic citizenship also refer to how HIV has been able to 'stitch together such apparently disparate phenomena as condom demonstrations, CD4 counts, sexual empowerment, retroviral genotyping, an ethic of sexual responsibility, and compliance with complex drug regimens, into a remarkably stable worldwide formation' (ibid.: 126). As Nguyen puts it, 'therapeutic citizenship is a biopolitical citizenship, a system of claims and ethical projects that arise out of the conjunction of techniques used to govern populations and manage individual bodies' (ibid.).

and contributed towards the emergence of a new AIDS activist movement in South Africa.

Conventional theories about rights-based social movements tend to posit instrumental rationality and individual rational choice as the rationale for participation. Critics of this approach claim that rights talk generally contributes towards depoliticisation, individualisation and the proverbial 'end of politics' (see Chapter 1). Such theories cannot, however, adequately account for how the structural conditions of marginality, the political culture of the anti-apartheid struggle, and experiences of illness and treatment have contributed towards the formation and everyday practices of organisations such as TAC. Neither can these theories adequately account for how the experience of illness and spoiled identities associated with AIDS stigma, denial and discrimination are reconfigured and transformed by TAC activists into a badge of pride, a new HIV-positive identity and form of social belonging. This new identity, I suggest, cannot be understood simply in terms of the instrumentalist logic of rights and political and legal struggles for access to health resources. Neither is this struggle for recognition and human dignity in the face of threats of stigma and social and biological death necessarily confined to hyper-marginalised members of society. This perhaps explains why, although the majority of its members are working-class or unemployed, TAC also appeals to HIV-positive middle-class students and professionals. The organisation's appeal has also spread to (HIV-negative) human rights activists and ordinary citizens who see in TAC's leadership and mobilisation strategies a heroic and progressive vision of 'moral truth' and social justice. Clearly TAC is able to articulate commonalities across a range of differences in ways that resemble the multi-class, multi-ethnic and non-racial composition of the United Democratic Front (UDF), an anti-apartheid umbrella organisation that emerged in South Africa in the mid-1980s. Notwithstanding the extraordinary successes of TAC, it appears that the majority of HIV-positive South Africans prefer to avoid joining an organisation that encourages, if not obliges, its HIV-positive members to publicly disclose their status. This may also explain why relatively few HIV-positive people who use private health care are willing to wear the HIV-positive T-shirt and 'out' themselves.

Like the Slum Dwellers International (SDI) activists who argue that they are concerned with much more than housing (see Chapter 4), MSF and TAC activists claim that they provide much more than AIDS drugs, condoms and the promise of a more equitable access to health care. They also provide the possibility of meaning and human dignity for people facing a profoundly stigmatising and lethal pandemic. To reduce TAC and MSF to a rights-based movement solely concerned with access to health resources underestimates the movement's work at the level of the body, subjectivity and identity. Neither can mainstream social movement theory account for the powerful ways in which activists with HIV/AIDS make meaning of their terrifying and traumatising journeys from the shadow of death to 'new life'. It is in this passage from the space of social and biological death that Turner's analysis of the ritual process can illuminate how new HIV-statuses, political subjectivities and convictions are rooted and routinised.

Some concluding thoughts on 'biological citizens' and 'responsibilised subjects'

Rights-based struggles for health care have increasingly become catalysts for the production of new forms of biomedical citizenship. For example, Adriana Petryna (2002) writes about how, following the Chernobyl disaster, the newly independent Ukrainian state, radiation research clinics and NGOs 'mediated an informal economy of illness and claims' that she refers to as 'biological citizenship'. This new form of citizenship involved selective access to social welfare based on scientific and legal criteria that both acknowledge injury and provide compensation for it. These struggles for biological citizenship unfolded in a context of the failure of the Ukrainian state to address massive unemployment, inflation and pervasive corruption. Within this context sufferers became dependent on being able to make 'claims for biomedical resources, social equity, and human rights' (Petryna, 2002: 192). Similarly, unemployed and poverty-stricken South Africans draw on the scientific language of CD4 counts and viral loads in order to access the disability grants provided to HIV-positive citizens with CD4 counts below 200. It was also reported in the press that some poor and unemployed citizens are consciously infecting themselves, or threatening to stop treatment, in order to access this R780 per month disability grant. These are examples of the ways in which, in places such as the Ukraine and South Africa, relationships between citizens and the state are being redefined in the course of life-and-death struggles over access to health care and social welfare. Another example is the TAC's Constitutional Court challenge that compelled the South African Government to provide Nevirapine to pregnant mothers as part of a national prevention of mother-to-child transmission (PMTCT) programme.

AIDS activism in South Africa has also contributed towards new forms of health citizenship that are concerned with both rights-based struggles and creating collectively shared meanings of the extreme experiences of illness and stigmatisation of individual AIDS sufferers. Drawing on the successes of MSF treatment programmes and TAC treatment literacy campaigns in Khayelitsha and Lusikisiki, public health professionals have called for the creation of an empowered citizenry with high levels of understanding of AIDS issues reinforced by community advocacy and mobilisation processes that promote the rights of people living with HIV/AIDS. According to the David Coetzee and Helen Schneider (2004: 1), a 'public health revolution' is necessary if ART is to succeed:

> Alternative approaches to the traditional management of chronic diseases, such as 'directly observed therapy', are needed if the stringent adherence requirements of ART are to be achieved. The evidence from pilot projects is that high levels of adherence stem from 'a new kind of contract between providers and clients'. The contract is premised on very high levels of understanding, treatment literacy and preparation on the part of users, the establishment of explicit support systems around users, and community advocacy processes that promote the rights of people living with HIV/AIDS. The responsibility for adherence is given to the client within a clear framework of empowerment and support. This is very different to the traditional

> paternalistic and passive relationship between health care workers and patients – changing this represents the key innovation challenge of an ART programme.
>
> (Coetzee and Schneider 2004: 72–3)

The idea of a contract – written or unwritten – between providers and clients is not new in the public health field. However, the nature and scale of the AIDS pandemic, along with the requirement of life-long treatment, reinvigorated calls for a change in the paternalistic culture associated with conventional public health interventions. These calls took place in a context in which the national health minister had conceded that DOT-TB programmes were failing, largely because of 'insufficient human resources to supervise and monitor implementation'. This had resulted in a declining cure rate for TB of only 53 per cent (*Cape Times*, 12 October 2004). In the terms of this call for a paradigm shift, clients would be entitled to free government health care, including antiretroviral drugs, but they would also need to demonstrate that they were 'responsibilised clients', through treatment adherence, disclosing their HIV status, using condoms, abstaining from alcohol abuse and smoking, and having healthy diets and lifestyles.

'Responsibilisation' also appears in political theorists' writings about contemporary liberal rationalities of government in the UK and Europe. For example, Barry *et al.* (1996) use the term to refer to the ways in which, under contemporary versions of liberalism, UK citizens are encouraged to govern themselves. Instead of burdening the National Health Service (NHS), they ought to take care of themselves and become responsible for health issues previously held to be the responsibility of the state. South African public health professionals and activists are calling for something different. They argue that what is needed for AIDS treatment and prevention programmes to succeed is a well-resourced and responsive public sector health system *and* empowered, knowledgeable and 'responsibilised' client-citizens. They are calling for an effective health system together with new forms of community participation and citizenship, or what Arjun Appadurai (2001) describes as auto-governmentality or 'governance from below'.

Phumzile Nywagi's testimony reveals that HIV illness and treatment experiences are often narrated in ways that reveal hybrid subjectivities and multiple interpretative frames, including religious, communal, biomedical and liberal modernist rights-based discourses. This suggests that the 'responsibilised' and empowered citizen-patient that public health professionals desire may not be simply a product of modern, liberal individualist conceptions of the rights-bearing citizen. It is for this reason that Turner's analysis of the ritual process can serve as a useful heuristic device for producing a more complex and nuanced understanding of illness and treatment experiences. Turner's approach suggests that the transformation into a 'responsibilised citizen' is the product of more than HIV/AIDS awareness campaigns, sex education, treatment literacy and rational choice. It is animated by the transformational (ritual) process of progressing from 'near death' to 'new life.'

Phumzile's testimony also reveals how a creative combination of religious, communal and activist mediations and interpretations of these traumatic transitions can, under certain conditions, contribute towards the conversion of HIV-positive people into committed activists and responsibilised citizens. However, AIDS activists, like any other social actors, are able to shift discursive and narrative frames depending on the specific context and audience. For instance, the illness experience/personal transformation frame may appear in testimonies in a particular form when used to rally others collectively, while shifting again into the more abstract and generic responsibilised citizen frame in interactions with patients at clinics, treatment literacy audiences, MSF staff, public health professionals and policy makers and so on. Social movement theories are generally incapable of appreciating the fluid and situational character of these discursive framings and the complex ways in which these are deployed in social movements. Finally, the moral politics of AIDS discussed in this chapter has produced collectively shared meanings and forms of political subjectivity and citizenship that have transformed representations of the Third World AIDS victim-sufferer as *homo sacer*, the Roman law figure who could be killed but not sacrificed.

The following chapter describes how Phumzile Nywagi, having survived this journey from 'near death' to 'new life', went on to establish Khululeka, a HIV men's support group in Gugulethu, Cape Town. It focuses on Khululeka's attempts to reconstitute the lives of its members after HIV diagnosis and treatment. The chapter describes how this process involved engaging with questions of masculinity and social reproduction in a post-apartheid setting characterised by competing traditions of constitutional democracy and deeply entrenched cultures of patriarchy, another clash between rights and culture.

7

Sexual Rights & Sexual Cultures
AIDS Activism, Sexual Politics & 'New Masculinities' after Apartheid[1]

Introduction

The AIDS pandemic in South Africa has contributed towards prising open questions on sexuality and sexual rights in ways that were unprecedented in the past. Partly as a result of exposure to HIV/AIDS prevention programmes driven by the international health agencies, the state, NGOs and social movements such as the Treatment Action Campaign (TAC), parents and politicians are increasingly compelled to talk openly about sex and sexual rights in the home and in public domains. Meanwhile gender, gay, AIDS and anti-rape activists have responded to the pandemic by highlighting the need to activate and realise the gender and sexual rights provisions in South Africa's progressive constitution. However, the AIDS pandemic and the promotion of new sexual and gender rights has also triggered a conservative backlash from religious leaders and 'traditionalists'. It is within this contested setting that new forms of AIDS activism and sexual citizenship are emerging.

Modern democracies everywhere are increasingly concerned with questions of sexual equality between homosexuals and heterosexuals, as well as between men and women (Fassin 2006). 'The politicisation of sexuality', Eric Fassin concludes, 'partakes in a broader process of denaturalisation of the social order [and is] therefore an object of democratic debate ... This is why sex is the [latest] frontier in the democratic definition of our societies' (ibid.: 92). In South Africa, the AIDS pandemic, same-sex marriages legislation, gender equity policies, and high profile sexual harassment cases all contributed towards the *sexualisation of politics and the politicisation of sexuality*. In 2006 the media reported on a number of high profile sex scandals that involved senior politicians and government officials. The expulsion of former African National Congress (ANC) chief whip Mbulelo Goniwe from parliament and party structures in 2006 appeared to signal a zero tolerance

---

[1] I would like to thank Jean Comaroff, Chris Colvin and the anonymous JSAS reviewers for their insightful comments on earlier drafts of this paper. I would also like to thank Manmeet Bindra, Phumzile Nywagi and members of Khululeka for their support and insights.

144

policy towards sexual harassment. It also signalled the growing influence of gender and sexual equality activism within the ANC. The ANC government's promotion of same sex marriage legislation in 2006 in the face of strong conservative opposition was another indication that sexual equality was becoming a new frontier of democratisation in post-apartheid South Africa.

This chapter will focus on these post-apartheid sexual developments in relation to, firstly, the sexual politics that surrounded the 2006 rape trial of the former deputy president Jacob Zuma, and secondly the establishment by Phumzile Nywagi, a former TAC and MSF activist, of Khululeka, a community-based HIV men's support group in Gugulethu, Cape Town. These two cases, it will be argued, reflect new forms of sexual politics that highlight contested interpretations of rights, morality, religion, culture and political leadership. They also serve as a mirror onto the tension between sexual rights and patriarchal cultures. Social movements, NGOs and community-based initiatives such as TAC and Khululeka have to constantly navigate their way through this highly contested terrain.

Whereas race and class dominated oppositional politics during the apartheid era, sexual and gender rights now compete for space in the post-apartheid public sphere. There is a glaring gap, however, between the progressive character of official state, constitutional and NGO endorsements of gender and sexual equality on the one hand, and the deeply embedded ideas and practices that reproduce gender and sexual inequality on the other. Idealised conceptions of civil society – often shared by the elite educated middle classes, including activists, academics, NGOs, and journalists – generally fail to adequately acknowledge its unruly and uncivil character.[2]

The discussion is divided into two sections. The first section focuses on the contested nature of the sexual politics that surrounded the Jacob Zuma rape trial, and highlights the responses of Zuma supporters, NGOs, activists and journalists. It shows how these responses reveal a deep-seated clash between the sexual and gender equality ideals enshrined in the constitution and promoted by progressive civil society organisations, and the sexual conservatism of Zuma's supporters and the broader public. This section also focuses on how ideas about traditional Zulu masculinity were represented and performed in the Zuma trial, thereby highlighting a tension between constitutional conceptions of universalistic sexual rights on the one hand, and particularistic sexual cultures on the other. This tension, I argue, is reproduced through the rhetorical productivity of a series of binaries: modern and traditional, rights and culture, liberal democracy and African communitarianism. This conflict of values was also evident in media and popular responses to the Zuma rape trial, including activist mobilisations, and public debates on political leadership and sexual rights. The section concludes by locating discourses on hegemonic masculinities within the context of the political and moral economy of sex in contemporary South Africa.

---

[2]   The Zuma rape trial drew attention to the complexities, internal contradictions and tensions within an African National Congress (ANC) ruling party and government that is committed to a progressive, rights-based constitutional democracy whilst having to accommodate and placate strategic allies, leadership figures and rank-and-file members who endorse social conservatism alongside their political radicalism. The Zuma Affair, it would seem, stretched this politics of moderation and accommodation to its limits.

The second section is concerned with innovative attempts by a group of young men in Cape Town to create 'alternative masculinities' (Connell 1996) in a time of AIDS. It focuses on Khululeka, a Cape Town township-based support group for men living with AIDS. Khululeka is an offshoot from the AIDS social movement Treatment Action Campaign (TAC). It was formed largely in response to the belief of its founder, Phumzile Nywagi, that township men were conspicuously absent from public clinics and HIV/AIDS support groups. Whereas TAC tends to be a predominantly rights-based movement largely comprising women, Khululeka has attempted to address men's issues, including dominant male sexual cultures. It has sought to fashion new alternative masculinities at a time when African men are increasingly singled out in the media and popular discourse as the source of sexual violence and HIV infection. Rather than romanticising these interrogations of traditionalist masculinities and portraying them as heroic counter-hegemonic forms of resistance from below, a close reading of the accounts of Khululeka members reveals ambivalent responses to these hegemonic masculinities. This suggests that the Khululeka case, like the other case studies in this book, challenges the binaries of modern and traditional, rights and culture, liberalism and communitarianism. The Khululeka case also raises a number of other questions. For instance, how different are these reconstructions of dominant masculinities and calls for 'sexual responsibility' from those promoted by public health professionals, global health agencies, religious conservatives and traditionalists? What are the implications of these discourses on sexuality for responding to HIV/AIDS and for furthering our understandings of post-apartheid politics, sexual rights, citizenship, and liberal democracy?

Situating sexual politics after apartheid
Same-sex marriage laws and anti-sexist legislation, as well as provisions to protect the rights of women, gay and lesbian citizens and people living with AIDS, are all by-products of South Africa's progressive constitutional democracy. The constitution, together with grassroots activism, has also contributed towards generating new forms of sexual politics in which concepts such as misogyny, patriarchy, sexism, homophobia and harassment have entered into mainstream public discourse. Meanwhile, social movements such as the Treatment Action Campaign (TAC), as well as public health professionals, NGOs and researchers, have highlighted the importance of gender equality and sexual rights and responsibilities in the fight against HIV/AIDS. However, these rights-based advances in the name of sexual and gender equality have also been catalysts for a conservative backlash in South Africa. These developments suggest that state and civil society advocates of these rights constitute a relatively small, educated, middle-class enclave within a sea of sexual conservatism. Like the legalisation of abortion and the abolition of the death penalty, sexual equality provisions such as same-sex marriage would probably be banished were they to be put to a referendum.

This brand of conservatism is of course not uniquely South African. Whereas in South Africa sexual conservatism is promoted and defended by the populace in the face of progressive state legislation, in the United States it was President George W. Bush and his faith-based administration who sought to banish same-sex marriage laws and HIV/AIDS prevention initiatives that promote condoms and sexual education.[3] In response to the internationalisation of gender and sexual rights programmes, the Bush Administration systematically cut the funding of domestic and global health programmes involving abortion and condom distribution. These faith-based interventions reflect an attempt by religious conservatives to prevent what they perceive to be the erosion of traditional Christian family values.[4] In addition to these examples of faith-based conservatism, global AIDS and sexual health programmes have also encountered widespread questioning of both sexual rights discourses and biomedical explanations of HIV/AIDS. These challenges to global health interventions raise questions about the sweeping claims of critical theorists of biomedicine who, following Foucault, have stressed the all-encompassing nature of the regulatory and disciplinary aspects of medicine and public health programmes (Adams and Pigg 2005; Singer 1990; Turner 1992).[5] They also raise questions about the ability of NGOs, social movements and activists to mediate these new forms of sexual citizenship.

This chapter focuses specifically on the contested character of sexual rights discourses that have been introduced by a post-apartheid state and mediated by NGOs, social movements and community activists. Whereas Chapters 5 and 6 focused on the role of social movements and NGOs in promoting health citizenship in relation to ARV treatment, section two of this chapter is concerned with a community-based initiative that attempts to mediate new forms of 'responsibilised masculinity' in contexts characterised by deeply embedded cultures of patriarchy and 'traditional

---

[3] See Garry Wills, 'Bush's Faith-Based Government', *The New York Review of Books*, 16 November 2006, p. 10. Wills notes that, in a show of support for his evangelical constituency, President Bush ensured that $170 million were made available for promoting a policy of 'abstinence only' in US schools during 2005. Meanwhile, the Centre of Disease Control removed from its website the findings of a panel that abstinence-only programmes do not work, and 30% of Bush's $15 billion Presidential Programme for AIDS Relief (PEPFAR) to prevent and treat AIDS in Africa was earmarked for promoting sexual abstinence and none of it was for condoms. This directly challenges the A (Abstinence), B (Be faithful) and C (Condomise) approach of mainstream AIDS prevention programmes by seeking to exclude the 'C' of ABC.

[4] In *Erotic Welfare: Sexual Theory and Politics in the Age of Epidemic*, Linda Singer (1990) writes that AIDS contributed towards the emergence of *a logic of contagion*, 'a panic logic' that profoundly influenced political and cultural life in the United States in the 1980s and 1990s. Singer identifies this 'panic logic' in numerous domains, including 'outbreaks' of new 'epidemics' such as teenage pregnancy, child abuse, rape, and drug abuse. This epidemic logic, Singer argues, was accompanied by heightened forms of sexual regulation and adversely impacted upon women's attempts to achieve 'reproductive freedom' and challenge the hegemony of the nuclear family. This 'panic logic' also contributed to increasing public calls for regulatory practices such as mandatory AIDS testing, quarantining those who are HIV-positive, and mandatory notification of sexual partners. Alongside these conservative calls to arms, there was a heightened religious and New Right rhetoric on 'family values' and the immorality of homosexuality. There were also calls for constitutional amendments against abortion, cutbacks on sex education and contraception, and popular opposition to the development of reproductive technologies These developments are interpreted by Singer as part of a conservative backlash against the 'sexual revolution' of the 1960s-1970s in the United States.

[5] Vincanne Adams and Stacey Leigh Pigg (2005) deploy a Foucaultian critique of public health in developing their argument that the recent proliferation of sex education and sexual health programmes in the Global South, largely in response to the AIDS pandemic, has strengthened surveillance medicine's capacity and contributed towards the global expansion of processes of the 'medicalisation,' 'scientisation' and 'normalisation' of sexuality and sexual health (Adams and Pigg. 2005: 26). They argue that, for the past few decades, millions of people all over the world have been exposed to public health programmes and workshops, manuals, pamphlets and curricula material on family planning, reproductive health, STDs, HIV/AIDS awareness, and sexual health. As a result, a relatively standardised and universalised body of medico-scientific knowledge on 'sexuality', sexual health and disease has been disseminated on a global scale.

masculinities'. The discussion of the sexual politics surrounding the Zuma rape trial suggests that whereas gender and sexual equality is enshrined in the South African Constitution, promoted by the political leadership and civil society organisations, and embraced by certain sections of the public, the claiming of these rights has generated a groundswell of conservative opposition in the broader society. This does not mean, however, that local communities have completely rejected rights-based discourses. Instead, it is the claiming of specific gender and sexual rights – for instance same-sex marriage – that has produced such profound discomfort and opposition amongst many South Africans. Contrary to idealised conceptions of civil society as a virtuous space of liberal democratic values, South African civil society, as in other parts of the world, is a highly contested, contradictory and ambiguous space.

Opposition to same-sex marriage was also evident in the responses of some members of the ANC political leadership. For example, speaking at Heritage Day celebrations in KwaZulu-Natal province on 24 September 2006, former deputy president Jacob Zuma told a large crowd of supporters that: 'When I was growing up an *ungqingili* (a gay) would not have stood in front of me. I would knock him out.' Zuma was also quoted as saying that same-sex marriages were 'a disgrace to the nation and to God'.[6] Yet, as a result of an avalanche of criticism from human rights and gay and lesbian activists, Zuma apologised for his statements, saying that the 'Constitution clearly states that nobody should be discriminated against on any grounds, including sexual orientation, and I uphold and abide by the Constitution of our land'.[7] Zuma's response reflected his own ambivalence and unease in relation to the tensions between sexual rights and sexual culture. These tensions are also part of the political landscape within which social movements, NGOs and community activists operate.

The public participation debates surrounding the Civil Unions Bill also revealed widely held homophobic and patriarchal attitudes that were sanctioned and promoted by citizens and conservative religious, political and traditional leaders. For example, in October 2006 a conservative Christian group, the Marriage Alliance of South Africa, organised a march to the Union Buildings to deliver a memorandum opposing same-sex marriage. Opposition to the Civil Unions Bill also emanated from the Congress of Traditional Leaders (Contralesa). Contralesa incurred the wrath of gay activists by claiming that homosexuality, the Civil Unions Bill, and the recognition of same-sex marriage were fundamentally 'un-African'. Nonhlanhla Mkhize of the Durban gay and lesbian community and health centre responded by claiming that Contralesa's leaders were in denial about the existence of African lesbian and gay people: 'There is ample research illustrating African people have engaged in same-sex relationships throughout our history. For example, in Namibia, Kenya, Nigeria and South Africa, bond friendships, ancestral wives, female husbands and male wives have existed for centuries as forms of same-sex relationships. All these relationships were accepted and respected in Africa before colonialism and apartheid'.[8] Gay activists were outraged by the overt hostility to

---

6   *Mail & Guardian*, 26 September 2006.
7   Ibid.
8   Angela Quintal, 'Gays attack traditional leaders: "Stop saying homosexual activities are unAfrican"', *Cape Times*, 27 October 2006, p.5.

same-sex marriage and gay rights exposed at these public hearings. For instance, Jonathan Berger, a lawyer from AIDS Law Project (ALP), in his submission to the home affairs parliamentary portfolio committee on the Civil Unions Bill, noted that 'the atmosphere [at the hearings] generally was extremely homophobic'.[9] Portfolio committee members had asked people who appeared before the committee questions such as 'What is gay?', 'How do two men have sex with each other?' and 'How do two women have a baby together?'.[10]

The hearings revealed a chasm between progressive sexual rights and conservative public reactions.[11] They also revealed that, although NGOs and civil society organisations were vocal and visible in the public sphere, in South Africa, as in many other parts of the Global South, their members appeared to be largely confined to the relatively small elite enclave of the educated middle classes (Chatterjee 2004). Similarly, while social movement, NGO and public health responses to the AIDS pandemic may have contributed towards a 'sexual revolution' in terms of which formerly taboo topics on sex have morphed into morally respectable subjects for discussion and debate in both private and public spaces, this had not translated into the realisation of the sexual and gender equality as envisaged by the architects of the constitution. Far from romanticising civil society as a space of grassroots democracy, AIDS and gender activists viewed the Zuma trial as a disturbing lens onto sexist and authoritarian tendencies within South Africa's '(un) civil society'. While progressive NGOs and civil society organisations such as the TAC and MSF have had considerable success and visibility in their struggles to promote sexual and gender equality and health citizenship, they have also had to confront deeply conservative sexual ideas and practices.

Section 1 – 'The Zuma Affair': A lens onto hegemonic masculinities?

In a context of entrenched patriarchal cultures, conservative religious movements, HIV/AIDS and extraordinarily high levels of sexual violence and rape, it is perhaps not surprising that the promotion of sexual rights has provoked such heated debate. The rise of AIDS, gay and gender activism has contributed towards transforming private sexual matters into contested public concerns. In addition, like the United States and other parts of the world, a conservative reaction to this sexual revolution is being fuelled by the rise of Evangelical Christianity and the promotion of moralising discourses on family values. In South Africa, this backlash has also been fuelled by President Thabo Mbeki's promotion of gender equality within ANC party and government structures. These calls for gender and sexual equality have catalysed a conservative mobilisation and re-articulation of deeply embedded discourses on African tradition and Christian family values.

---

[9] *Mail & Guardian*, 20 October, p .23.

[10] Ibid.

[11] The disjuncture between constitutionally enshrined sexual rights and everyday gendered realities is also evident in the extraordinarily high incidence of rape and sexual violence in South African society. For example, it is estimated that at least one in three South African women will be raped in her lifetime (see Moffett, 2006: 129).

This clash of values around sexuality was very evident during Jacob Zuma's rape trial in May 2006. During the trial, which was held in the Johannesburg High Court, the former deputy president and his defence counsel argued that the rape accuser had seduced Zuma by wearing 'revealing clothes' (See Zapiro cartoon, p. xvi). The clothing referred to here was the kanga, a traditional African cloth that is worn in villages throughout the sub-continent. As *Mail & Guardian* reporter Nicole Johnston pointed out the African kanga 'has been the hallmark of female modesty and respectability [and is] handed out at political rallies emblazoned with slogans and the faces of political leaders' (*Mail & Guardian*, 5 May 2006, p. 2). During the trial, however, the mundane cotton kanga was sexualised and transformed into an object of seduction, much like the infamous cigar during the Monica Lewinsky and Bill Clinton scandal. Responding to what they perceived to be a systematic attempt to discredit the rape accuser and portray her as an unscrupulous seducer, a small group of gender and anti-rape activists from the People Opposing Women Abuse (POWA) faced a huge crowd of jeering Zuma supporters when they demonstrated outside the Johannesburg High Court dressed in cotton kangas. As the journalist Johnston concluded, they were demonstrating to 're-appropriate their right to wear the kanga – anywhere, any time' (*Mail & Guardian*, 5 May 2006, p. 2).

Zuma was ultimately acquitted and the rape accuser was portrayed by Justice Willem van der Merwe as a manipulative seductress, a pathological liar and a serial rape accuser. The judge also lashed out at the media, activists and Zuma supporters for prejudging the case and being more interested in sexual and gender politics than the actual evidence presented in the rape case. The judge chastised pressure groups, NGOs, governmental organisations and the media for having 'breached the *sub judice* rule'. In the preface to his 174-page judgement delivered in the Johannesburg High Court on 4 May 2006, the judge argued that 'it is not acceptable that a court be bombarded with political, personal or group agendas and comments. As one contributor to a daily newspaper very correctly put [it]: "This trial is more about sexual politics and gender relations than it is about rape."' In his final concluding statement, the white judge also lambasted Zuma for having unprotected sex with an HIV-positive woman and being unable to control his sexual desires. Paraphrasing Kipling, Judge van der Merwe concluded, 'If you can control your sexual urges, then you are a man, my son'.[12] This statement revealed how lingering colonial legacies of racial paternalism continued to discursively link sex, gender and race in post-apartheid South Africa.

This moralising tone from the white judge, as well as similar utterances from other quarters including the media, NGOs and religious leaders, provoked angry responses from Zuma's supporters. In a public statement on 25 May 2006, Senzeni Zokwana, the president of the National Union of Mineworkers (NUM), attacked the hypocrisy of those who drew on 'Christian morality' to judge and condemn Zuma for his sexual behaviour. According to Zokwana, not all NUM's members were Christians, and not all of them adhered to the 'Ten Commandments', in particular the prohibition on adultery. This statement, made in a deeply Christian country,

---

[12] For the full judgement see the *Mail & Guardian* website: http://www.mg.co.za/specialreport.aspx?area =zuma_report.

unsurprisingly unleashed heated discussions on the Friends of Jacob Zuma (FJZ) website about the relationship between sexuality, morality, Christianity and the secular state.[13] Many pro-Zuma website contributors belonging to the trade union movement, the SACP and ANC and Communist Party youth leagues supported Zokwana's statement, and portrayed Zuma as a 'man of the people', a heroic fighter for the liberation of the black working class, the downtrodden and destitute. 'Lekua', a vehemently pro-Zuma contributor to the website, defended Zuma's moral integrity, and Zokwana's statement, in a posting on 25 May 2006:

> On the selective morality, namely that it is alright for a woman to lay a false rape charge but it is uncalled for JZ to have breached his marriage vows, NUM [Zokwana] said: "NUM does not subscribe to the Ten Commandments, especially the one that says "Thou shall not commit adultery."" This hardline stance by Cosatu and its largest affiliate, NUM, clearly shows that *the whole nation is getting impatient with the hypocrites* who behave as if they are hollier [sic] than JZ and all of us. *Their dictatorial tendencies has [sic] inspired the whole nation into action to reclaim the ANC from the elites and restore it to the masses* who are still poor and destitude [sic]. (my emphasis)[14]

Here we see how questions of sexual behaviour and religious morality were reconfigured into populist rhetoric on African nationalism and the need 'to reclaim the ANC from the elites and restore it to the masses'. These responses were set against the backdrop of bruising political battles between supporters of President Thabo Mbeki and former deputy president Zuma. Zuma's supporters comprised a mix of trade unionists, communists, ANC Youth League figures and Zulu neo-traditionalists. This powerful support base demanded that their leader should become the next president, notwithstanding President Mbeki's dismissal, in 2005, of Zuma from his position as deputy president. This followed the decision by the prosecuting authority to prosecute Zuma on corruption and, some months later, rape charges. These trials, as well as President Mbeki's calls for the next president to be a woman, were seen to be part of an elaborate anti-Zuma conspiracy orchestrated by the office of the president. The conspirators were also portrayed on the FJZ website as a part of President Mbeki's 'Xhosa nostra'. Postings on the website also claimed that President Mbeki wanted his female Xhosa-speaking deputy president, Phumzile Mlambo-Ngcuka, to succeed him in order to prevent Zuma becoming the next president:

> So the president has spoken the next president of RSA should be a 'woman'. And every one knows that 'woman' word read Ngcuka's wife [sic] ... According to the intelligent Mbeki all men are unproductive and all women are [productive]. When are we going to have a gay or lesbian president? At present I do not see any woman that is ready to rule this country.[15]

Zuma supporters were especially upset with President Mbeki's introduction of quotas for women in political office and ANC structures. Mbeki's ANC government was also perceived to be undermining the powers of traditional leaders through local government reform. Demonstrations outside the court included the presence of *iinyanga* (traditional healers) using herbal medicines to ensure that Zuma was

---

[13] See http://www.friendsofjz.co.za
[14] http://www.friendsofjz.co.za/viewmessage.asp
[15] Ndosi, 06/05/2006, http://www.friendsofjz.co.za/viewmessage.asp

successfully acquitted in his trial. Meanwhile *amakosi* (chiefs) dressed in traditional skins occupied the front seats of the courtroom during proceedings. The FJZ website also had hundreds of postings alleging plots perpetrated by Mbeki's inner circle, the media, big business, neo-liberals, and even Christians. These claims circulated in the media and on the FJZ website well after Zuma's acquittal on the rape charges.[16]

The Zuma rape trial became a key discursive site in an ongoing leadership struggle between Zuma's supporters, including the SACP and COSATU on the one side, and President Mbeki and his followers on the other. This leadership struggle split the ANC into two factions, those who supported Zuma's populist (and traditionalist) leadership style, and those who supported Mbeki's more centralist and managerialist democratic approach. This divide also coincided with deep ideological cleavages within the tripartite alliance of the ANC, COSATU and the SACP. From the perspective of COSATU and the SACP, President Mbeki's neo-liberal economic policies benefited big business and global capital rather than the workers. The ANC appeared to be split down the middle by ideological divisions and President Mbeki's leadership style. The sexual politics surrounding the rape trial provided a public space for the expression of these deep divides.

For media commentators and gender activists, the trial was a lens onto a deeply embedded authoritarian culture of patriarchy, misogyny, and sexual violence. However, few commentators reflected on the historical transformations that produced these cultural forms and social practices (see below). Instead, commentary was focused on the visceral immediacy of events inside and outside the court. For example, journalists covering the daily demonstrations outside the Johannesburg High Court reported on Zuma supporters who burnt photographs and effigies of the rape accuser and chanted 'burn the bitch'. Zuma's supporters, many of whom wore '100% Zulu Boy' T-shirts, were also accused of intimidating anti-rape activists protesting outside the court. The latter had launched a 'One in Nine Campaign' to draw attention to the fact that so few women are prepared to report their rapes to the police. Rape activists highlighted the fact that there were 55,000 reported cases of rape in 2004/05 whereas the South African Law Reform Commission had provided estimates of 1.69 million rapes per year.[17] Gender activists also questioned the judge's decision to permit the defence to lead testimony on the complainant's sexual history, a decision that activists believed was designed to demonstrate that she had a history of false rape accusations going back to her childhood. The judge demolished the complainant's evidence and endorsed Zuma's claim that he had

---

[16] These vociferous website responses to the rape trial were clearly more than simply clashes of moral values around sex and sexual equality. Instead, sexually conservative responses could be analysed as reflections of deep structural changes in the economy and society, e.g., global economic processes contributed towards the increasing devaluation and redundancy of male unskilled labour in South Africa. The rhetorical productivity of 'sex talk' often lies in its extraordinary capacity to allegorically link and condense anxieties about sex, the economy, politics and social reproduction. Anxieties about sex and family values in particular can be deciphered as popular commentaries on the radical ruptures of contemporary (neoliberal) capitalism and processes of social, economic and political transformation, especially male marginalisation. In other words, 'sex talk' surrounding the Zuma Affair can be analysed as a discursive site for reflecting upon historical transformations taking place in post-apartheid South Africa (see below).

[17] *Sunday Independent*, 16 April 2006.

consensual sex at his home in November 2005. Activists argued in the press that the treatment meted out to Zuma's rape accuser by both the judge and Zuma's supporters would simply reinforce this 'one in nine' syndrome amongst rape victims.

After the judgement against the 'kanga-clad seductress', gender activists appeared to have even stronger grounds for believing the judicial system would continue to be perceived by rape victims as unsympathetic to their predicament. Some activists also claimed that the relentless cross-examination of the complainant by Zuma's defence lawyer constituted 'secondary rape' of the victim by the criminal justice system. Zuma's acquittal, they argued, would also be interpreted by many of his followers as vindication of their patriarchal beliefs and claims that women are predisposed to fabricate rape in order to access money and power.

It was not only the gender activists who were enraged by Zuma's sexual behaviour. Zuma had also angered AIDS activists with his court testimony that he had sex without a condom with an HIV-positive woman because he had calculated that the risk of infection was low. Zuma also told the court that by showering after he had sex with the rape accuser he intended to reduce the risk of infection (See Zapiro cartoon, p. xiv). According to AIDS activists, these statements contributed towards widespread confusion and misinformation about HIV/AIDS, including the proliferation of AIDS myths, dissident theories, and popular beliefs that sex with virgins could cure AIDS and that the disease was caused by witchcraft. In his press conference a day after the acquittal Zuma apologised for having made a 'mistake' by having 'unsafe sex' with an HIV-positive woman. He stated that he would recommit himself to promoting AIDS prevention programmes. Yet, he still sought to justify his shower statement by telling a female journalist, 'If you've been in the kitchen, my dear, peeling onions, you wash your hands, not so? What's so funny about washing my hands after doing something?'[18]

Gender and AIDS activists and media commentators argued that Zuma's trial highlighted the deeply entrenched character of patriarchy in South African society. They also claimed that the trial reflected the dismal failure of the national political leadership to confront sexual violence and HIV/AIDS. After all, Zuma had been the president of both the Moral Regeneration Campaign and the South African National AIDS Commission (SANAC), government bodies that activists regarded as entirely ineffectual (See Zapiro cartoon, pp xiv and xv). These failures of government were perceived to be especially disturbing in a country with a 'rape pandemic' and an estimated 5.6 million people living with AIDS.[19] So, notwithstanding a progressive constitution that promised sexual rights and gender equality, as well as better health care for all, there seemed to be deeply embedded social and cultural barriers in the way of realising these rights.

---

[18] *Mail & Guardian*, 12 May 2006, p. 31.

[19] AIDS activists slammed the national leadership for a series of failures including President Mbeki's controversial denial of the scale of the pandemic, his questioning of the link between HIV and AIDS, and his support for dissident claims that antiretroviral drugs (ARVs) were dangerously toxic (see Robins, 2004). Similarly, the minister of health had infuriated AIDS activists by supporting the dubious AIDS remedies of vitamin manufacturer Dr Matthias Rath and promoting her own 'African solution' for AIDS comprising a diet of garlic, onion, the African potato and olive oil. Zuma's sexual behaviour and court statements were, from the perspective of activists, yet another leadership blunder.

Performing 'Zulu manhood': sexual rights versus sexual cultures?
During the liberation struggle questions of sexuality and sexual rights were gener-ally sidelined and subordinated within anti-apartheid political discourse. By 2006 this had significantly changed, and sexual politics seemed to be on the rise. Judge van der Merwe claimed that the Zuma rape trial had been transformed into a public drama about sexual politics. The trial was also transformed by the media into a morality tale that ended up reinforcing racist stereotypes about sexually irresponsible African men. Such representations of African sexuality had been vehemently contested by President Mbeki. In fact, the President's AIDS denialism seems to have been fuelled by his belief that AIDS and anti-rape activism rein-forced racist western ideas about promiscuous and disorderly African sexualities (see Chapter 5). This was also evident in President Mbeki's attack on the anti-rape activist Charlene Smith. In his weekly letter posted on the *ANC Today website*, the President claimed that Smith's commentary on South Africa's shocking rape statistics reproduced racist stereotypes of black men as habitual rapists. A similar attack was launched by ANC portfolio committee members against filmmaker Cliff Bestall for producing a devastating television documentary on baby rape. Although these troubling questions about African sexuality had been vigorously challenged by the president and ANC national leadership, the Jacob Zuma rape trial appeared to re-insert sexuality and masculinity squarely within the public domain.

In the Johannesburg High Court in May 2006, South Africans witnessed a tele-vised postmodern spectacle in which a tribal elder-cum-liberation struggle icon performed 'Zulu traditional masculinity' for consumption by both the court and the broader citizenry. According to Zuma's version of African masculinity, in Zulu culture 'leaving a woman in that state [of sexual arousal]' was the worst thing a man could do. 'She could even have you arrested and charged with rape', he told the attentive court. In other words, he would have violated and disrespected her had he not had sexual intercourse with her. Addressing the judge as *'nkosi' – yenkantolo* (the king of the court), Zuma referred to his accuser's private parts as *isibhaya sika bab'wakhe* (her father's kraal). He conceded that he entered 'the kraal' without *ijazi ka mkhwenyana* (the groom/husband's coat, i.e., a condom). These translations of isiZulu idioms are usually associated with deep rural KwaZulu-Natal. To those attending the Johannesburg High Court hearing, and millions of others following the trial through the extensive media coverage, these words signified that Zuma was indeed a 'real' Zulu man: '100% Zulu Boy' as his supporters' T-shirts put it. Here again, images of 'Zulu virility' seemed to represent and embody a broader post-apartheid political process of African retraditionalisation.

It was in his discussion of *lobola* (bridewealth) that Zuma publicly performed his 'Zulu masculinity' most vividly. In response to questions about two aunts who had attempted to initiate *lobola* negotiations with the complainant, Zuma answered that he 'had his cows ready'. As he put it, 'Lobola is an issue between the girl ... and the family. Should [Kwezi] have told these two ladies that "Yes, I want Zuma to pay lobola", I would definitely do it.' This discussion on *lobola* sought to valorise tradi-tional Zulu masculinity and thereby normalise and redeem his sexual behaviour.

Zuma's court statements suggested that he was indeed an authentic Zulu traditionalist. This representation of Zuluness was mediated to South Africans and the wider world via television, radio, the Internet and a local and international press fascinated with primordialist fantasies of Zulu culture. This representation of the '100% Zulu man' was strategic and effective in making the case that the sex had indeed been consensual. Zuma's behaviour was, after all, how Zulu men are meant to act, so this patriarchal argument went. This particular understanding of Zulu masculinity was self-consciously fashioned and situationally deployed by Zuma in the Johannesburg High Court as a sign of a revitalised Zulu traditionalism. It contrasted starkly with the image of President Mbeki as the (Xhosa) modernist architect of South Africa's rights-based constitutional democracy that is widely perceived to challenge African culture by undermining traditional leadership and promoting gender equity.

Zuma's performance of African masculinity was not that different to the ideas about Zuluness and customary law produced by Shepstone and countless other colonial officials. Historians and anthropologists have shown how these historical constructions of tradition and customary law were produced through ongoing conversations between colonial administrators and tribal elders (Channock 1985; Hamilton 1998; Mamdani 1996;). Zuma's version of Zulu masculinity performed at the Johannesburg High Court was packaged as primordial ethnic essence, and was designed to prop up Zuma's legal defence of consensual sex. This strategy was no doubt perceived by his legal team to be effective precisely because South Africa is a postcolonial country in which reified conceptions of African culture carry considerable clout in the courts and on the streets.

Zuma's performance of unblemished virile Zulu masculinity in court, as well as his homophobic comments at Heritage Day celebrations in September 2006, mirrored popular perspectives on sexuality, gender and masculinity. This also partly explains Zuma's popularity across a variety of constituencies, social classes and ideological camps including traditionalists, the ANC Youth League and the popular Left. For Zuma and his supporters within the SACP, ANC, and trade unions, being a 'traditional Zulu man' and a 'modern revolutionary' was neither contradictory nor incompatible. Zuma's popularity was precisely because of his ability to invent himself as a 'man for all seasons' and ideological persuasions, a post-ideological position that straddled the political binaries of Left and Right, modern and traditional. It also reflected the compatibility of political radicalism with social conservatism. What united Zuma's diverse constituency was the linking of African populism with traditional masculinity and conservative sexual politics. This traditional/modern binary was rhetorically and politically highly productive.

The following section interrogates this binary by drawing attention to transforming social and economic structures and how these have in turn influenced changing conceptions of African masculinity. This section questions timeless stereotypes of irresponsible, traditional African men by locating these masculinities within historical processes. It also deconstructs the ahistorical version of Zulu masculinity performed by Jacob Zuma in the Johannesburg High Court.

Historicising hegemonic masculinities and sexual conservatism

A South African Department of Health Report (2003) entitled *Men in HIV/AIDS Partnership: 'Men care enough to act'* reported on a series of consultative workshops in which men identified the following themes and strategies for tackling HIV/AIDS: unequal sexual and gender relations, culture and traditional values such as polygamy, *lobola* (bridewealth), virginity testing, gender stereotypes and masculinity. The workshops concluded that there was a need to embark upon education and awareness programmes that targeted young boys from the age of five to eighteen years in order to 'challenge the status quo and the men's world view' (ibid.: 11). Despite identifying these strategies and objectives, government programmes have done very little in terms of grappling with these questions of culture, identity and masculinity.

The report's ahistorical conception of 'African sexuality' ignores a growing literature on changing historical constructions of African masculinities and sexualities (Cornwall and Lindisfarne 1994; Delius and Glaser 2002; Heald 1995; Hunter 2006; Hoad *et al.* 2005; Moodie 1994; Mills and Ssewakiryanga 2005; Morrell 2001; Niehaus 2002; Ouzgane and Morrell 2005; Reid and Walker 2005; Richter and Morrell 2006;). Mark Hunter's (2006) work in rural KwaZulu Natal, for example, focuses on changes in the 'political economy of sex' that are partly responsible for fuelling the South Africa AIDS pandemic. Hunter challenges stereotypes that blame AIDS on African culture. He also questions political economy approaches that attribute the pandemic primarily to legacies of racial capitalism and apartheid and the destruction of African family structures through the system of circular male-migration. While not denying the historical role of apartheid in undermining African family structures, Hunter's work highlights relatively recent changes to the political economy of sex. He shows how, since the 1970s, dramatic changes in cultures of sexuality have occurred as a result of the combination of rising social inequalities, structural unemployment, greatly reduced marital rates and new forms of domestic and sexual fluidity (see Spiegel, 1995 on domestic fluidity). These developments have rendered both men and women more vulnerable. Studies suggest that the combination of male disempowerment and chronic poverty has, in certain cases, contributed towards aggressive male sexualities, which has in turn fuelled the spread of the pandemic (Hunter 2006; Wood and Jewkes 2001). These developments have also introduced changes in female sexuality, including forms of transactional sex for both survival and to support modern consumer lifestyles and identities (Hunter 2006; Leclerc-Madlala 2004).

Historians and anthropologists have also shown that in the past, in many parts of Africa, there were highly structured and culturally mediated ways in which young people were initiated into adulthood and adult forms of sexual activity (see Delius and Glaser 2002; Hunter 1979; Hunter 2006). For example, during the nineteenth century in parts of southern Africa, penetrative sex, fathering and fatherhood were linked to building a home (Hunter 2006). These cultural practices were subject to rapid and dramatic social change. In the early decades of the twentieth century, when increasing numbers of young men began to migrate to South African cities to search for work, they gained some independence in terms of *ilobola* payment. This allowed them to build their own families and homesteads without having to rely on their fathers' permission and help. However, with the decline of the migrant labour system since the 1970s it has becoming increasingly difficult for young men in Southern Africa to find permanent jobs. This era of structural unemployment has in turn made it extremely difficult for young men to pay *ilobola* and thereby get 'properly married'. These dramatic changes are of course not confined to South Africa but are being experienced acutely in many parts of sub-Saharan Africa. Yet, responses to these changing structural conditions of everyday life on the African continent are often interpreted and politicised through the lens of ahistorical stereotypes about a singular African sexuality.

Notwithstanding the economistic emphasis of Mark Hunter's (2006) study of the 'political economy of sex' – possibly to the neglect of questions of agency, desire and subjectivity – his work provides an important counterweight to the ahistorical representations of African sexuality that circulate in popular and public health discourses. These essentialist stereotypes of African masculinity and sexuality can be deployed for a variety of purposes. In the case of the Zuma rape trial, for instance, these ideas were deployed to normalise Zuma's sexual behaviour. For many men, including the modernist militants of the trade union movement and the popular Left, these traditionalist conceptions of African manhood were the bedrock of identity and belonging. The following section probes how these ideas, and alternatives to them, circulate in the lives of a group of men living with AIDS.

Section 2 – 'Brothers are doing it for themselves': alternative masculinities in a time of AIDS?

The Oscar-winning South African film *Tsotsi* tells the story of a fearless and violent township gangster who, as a young boy, ran away from home after his abusive father refused to let him near his mother who was dying of AIDS; the father believed that his son could be infected by touching his HIV-positive mother. One day Tstosi shoots a black woman while hijacking her car outside her middle-class suburban home. As he speeds off from the house in the woman's BMW he hears a baby crying in the back seat of the car. He eventually decides to take the baby to his township house and this dramatically changes his life. Through trying to care for the infant, Tsotsi goes on a 'road to Damascus' conversion process, and he decides to return the infant to its parents. The film ending hints that he decided to turn his back on crime and gangsterism. This redemptive storyline also suggests that even violent young men may be amenable to radical change and reform. It also hints that fatherhood can become a catalyst for the construction of new 'responsible masculinities' in the context of patriarchal cultures. This powerful cinematic narrative also contests popular and media images of young black men as the source of the problem of HIV/AIDS, domestic and sexual violence, rape and crime. The following section shows how Tsotsi's redemptive narrative resonates in certain respects with the stories of young men living with AIDS who have sought to transform their lives as a result of illness experiences and their recognition of the need to lead healthy and sexually responsible lifestyles and assume the 'proper' social roles of fatherhood.

Men behaving 'responsibly'

It is well documented that South African men tend to stay away from public health clinics, few get tested for HIV, and even fewer join AIDS support groups. When men do turn up at HIV, TB and STI clinics, they are often labelled by nurses and counsellors as the villains of the piece. They are blamed for being irresponsible in their sexual lives, health and lifestyles. Given that public health clinics are not known for being male-friendly, it is hardly surprising that clinics in South Africa remain largely women's spaces. This perhaps also explains why seven out of ten adults accessing antiretroviral therapy (ART) are women.

Notwithstanding the difficulties of integrating men into the public health system, they are increasingly being exposed to HIV prevention and treatment messages that call for responsible sex and lifestyles. This is especially the case for those men who test HIV-positive. For instance, HIV-positive patients have to meet a number of criteria to access antiretroviral therapy (ART). These selection criteria include disclosure of their status to at least one other individual, and participation in psychosocial counselling and peer support groups. Patients are also expected to refrain from consuming alcohol and drugs, and they have to agree to adhere to healthy diets, healthy lifestyles and drug adherence. These selection criteria can end up functioning as a form of social triage by screening out and excluding the poorest of the poor, especially unemployed men, who are more likely to be vulnerable to drug and alcohol abuse, and hence perceived to be less drug-adherent.

The Western Cape Province and MSF treatment programme in Khayalitsha, Cape Town, is an example of a donor-funded programme that has been able to produce exceptionally high levels of drug adherence. These programmes have also contributed towards profound transformations in patients' subjectivities and sexual lives (see above). These changes, which have been promoted through TAC community mobilisation and treatment literacy workshops, have contributed towards creating empowered, knowledgeable and drug-adherent patients. By March 2006, 16,234 people had passed through this ART programme in Khayelitsha. TAC and MSF also established a successful treatment programme in rural Lusikisiki (formerly Transkei) in the Eastern Cape Province. Many of the protocols and practices developed by MSF and TAC at these highly successful programmes have informed the national ART programme that commenced in April 2004. These kinds of community-based patient mobilisation programmes encourage new forms of therapeutic citizenship and responsibilised citizenship (see Chapter 6). The targets of these HIV prevention and treatment literacy programmes are required to develop new ways of caring for the self and being responsible in their sexual lives, diets and lifestyles (see Nguyen 2005).

A few years ago, Phumzile complained to me that Xhosa initiation rituals were no longer capable of teaching young men to act responsibly. This discussion emerged in the course of a number of discussions during which Phumzile told me about his youth, employment history, marriage and separation, his chronic illnesses as a result of HIV, and how he eventually joined the TAC and enrolled in an ARV programme at Khayelitsha, Cape Town. Reflecting on the role of initiation in an age of AIDS, Phumzile claimed that most young men returned from initiation as sexually irresponsible as they were before they went to 'the bush'.

> You know, initiation as it is, it doesn't mean anything nowadays. It's just pain, it seems. It doesn't give any way forward to life. One would just go to initiation for the sake of going there. But not knowing the concept traditionally, how our rituals [demand] that you have to change your lifestyle, to know yourself … One would go to initiation and come and do the same thing that he used to do. I mean there don't seem to be regulations around sex. I mean young people can sleep around with who they want. Or am I wrong? The church may say things, but do people listen? Parents may say one thing, but do they listen? Is there any authority, or is it the case that it's anarchic, and youth can do as they want?[20]

Phumzile's account of the failure of initiation stemmed from his frustration with counselling men about HIV prevention and treatment. He stated that he preferred counselling women as they, unlike men, took HIV seriously. Phumzile also told me about his own high risk sexual lifestyle and how he became ill as a result of HIV. Phumzile's illness and treatment experiences (see above) created the conditions for dramatic changes in his lifestyle. It also created the conditions for other changes in subjectivity, including his commitment to engaging with questions of responsible sexual behaviour and masculinity.

In September 2005, Phumzile established Khululeka Men's Support Group in Gugulethu, a working-class Xhosa-speaking township in Cape Town. *Khululeka* is a Xhosa word for 'freedom', 'to be free', or, as Phumzile put it, 'It means to feel free to talk about HIV.' The support group consists of a group of twenty young men, many of whom have participated in MSF and TAC antiretroviral (ARV) treatment (ART) programmes in Khayelitsha, Cape Town. It is one of a handful of HIV support groups in South Africa that focuses specifically on men's issues. Khululeka was started in response to Phumzile's observation that men were virtually invisible in community health clinics and AIDS support groups. All of the members of this group were open about their seropositive status, and their aim was to provide 'safe sex' education and treatment literacy in the communities in which they lived. In addition, since most of Khululeka's members were unemployed, the group wanted to develop opportunities for skills training and job creation.

The members of Khululeka regarded men as their primary target in their efforts to challenge AIDS stigma and promote healthy lifestyles and safe sex practices. They also address problems of unemployment, poverty, and HIV impacting on men's sense of identity and dignity. According to Phumzile, 'When you are HIV-positive, and on top of that you are unemployed, you can lose everything. Your wife and children don't respect you because you are sick, without a job, and now you cannot provide for them. You are nobody. You are useless. This is why we have created Khululeka, to help men discover their manhood and dignity again.' 'Themba', another Khululeka member stated the following: 'We saw that men were nowhere to be seen at support groups and clinics. They only visit clinics when they are seriously ill. They also sleep around, drink and smoke too much, and this is a problem

---

[20] Taped interview with Phumzile Nywagi, Cape Town, 1 September 2005.

when you take ARVs. This is why we decided we need to work with men.'

All of the members of Khululeka live openly with HIV, and they spoke about how disclosure allowed them to 'feel free,' and that this equipped them, both physically and psychologically, to deal with HIV and AIDS. According to 'Vuyo', 'HIV is just a mind game' and unless you develop the right psychological attitude you will be broken down and lose all strength and hope: 'HIV is just a mind game. But if you treat it like any other disease, like TB, then you can challenge it ... If you are diagnosed, your first thought is you will die. But now it is different – we have ARVs. Now behaviours need to change and so do our life styles.' Vuyo also referred to how illness could infantilise and undermine one's sense of manhood and dignity: 'My dreams vanished when I was diagnosed. When I was first diagnosed, I couldn't wash myself, walk or feed myself ... It was as if you are turned around back into being a baby.' It was this traumatic transition from being a healthy man to being a helpless 'baby' that rocked the existential foundations of Phumzile and Vuyo. These profoundly unsettling experiences destabilised their prior sense of self and identity. This extreme vulnerability facilitated the conditions for beginning a process of critical reflection on their pre-HIV lifestyles and identities, thereby creating the possibility of imagining new identities and ways of being in the world.

These radical changes in individual subjectivity and identity often accompanied a renewed commitment towards family, neighbours, and community, in particular in relation to fighting the pandemic. Khululeka was involved in numerous community-based activities, including AIDS awareness and sex education campaigns in public spaces such as township *shebeens* (taverns), railway stations and taxi ranks, on community radio talk shows, and at funerals of people who died of AIDS. They were also involved in collecting money for families that were unable to pay funeral costs, and visiting HIV-positive people in hospitals and their homes. The group's meeting place was a Rotary Club-funded shipping container in the backyard of Phumzile's house in Gugulethu. They had outings and *braais* (barbecues) where they socialised and discussed matters of common concern. These rituals of togetherness contributed towards the production of sociality under conditions of illness that are usually characterised by extreme stigma and social isolation.

Many of Khululeka's members carry the double burden of HIV/AIDS and structural unemployment.[21] Many also had children, but because of unemployment they were unable to formalise these relationships through marriage. One of the reasons

---

[21] Studies suggest that in the past young men stood a much better chance of gaining access to formal employment that allowed them to pay *ilobola* (bridewealth) and thereby marry, have children, and establish relatively stable family households. During the past three decades, however, dramatically rising rates of unemployment (currently estimated to be 30–40%) have made this life cycle trajectory increasingly difficult achieve. This has in turn undermined the ability of young men to assume the social roles of fatherhood. Mark Hunter (2006:106) observes that many Zulu-speaking men in KwaZulu-Natal are abandoning pregnant women because of conditions related to poverty and unemployment. Many of these men are extremely frustrated at not being able to conform to accepted social roles of fatherhood, including paying *inhlawulo* (damages for impregnation), *ilobolo* (bridewealth), and acting as a 'provider'. This creates conditions whereby manliness is partially boosted by fathering children, but at the same time those men who are unable to fulfil the social roles associated with fatherhood are branded as unmanly and 'irresponsible' (ibid.).

for the establishment of Khululeka was to address unemployment and thereby enhance the capacity of men to fulfil the social roles of fatherhood. Now that ARVs had given them their lives back, notwithstanding the long-term health uncertainties about living with HIV, they now had to reclaim their social lives, which in many cases had been put on hold as a result of illness. Finding a job was a crucial starting point in this production of 'new life'.

For Khululeka's members, being permanent volunteer TAC activists was no longer financially viable. Most of the men were between thirty and forty years old and were keen to establish stable families. Having managed to come to grips with their sero-positive status, and having accepted the reality of life-long commitment to ARV treatment, they turned their attention to new challenges. Whereas Phumzile envisaged that Khululeka members would seek out work as treatment literacy practitioners,[22] patient advocates and counsellors within the public health sector, it became apparent that they desired more conventionally masculinist forms of labour rather than working within a largely feminised health services sector. This expressed itself in the lack of interest amongst most Khululeka members for health-related training. It was therefore not surprising that by 2007 only two Khululeka members, both of whom had been trained as treatment literacy practitioners by TAC and MSF, had full-time employment.

Illness narratives, treatment testimonies and 'new' masculinities

For ARV and HIV prevention programmes to succeed it is necessary to have both a well-run and responsive public sector health system and empowered, knowledgeable and 'responsibilised' client-citizens. Public health professionals and activists are in fact calling for an effective health system together with new forms of community participation and citizenship, or what Arjun Appadurai (2001) describes as 'governance from below'. It is these concerns that are at the heart of the focus of MSF, TAC and Khululeka on innovative community-based initiatives in sex education, treatment literacy and social and economic support for people living with AIDS. These approaches have created the conditions for the emergence of new social identities, including the 'new masculinities' that seem to be emerging as a result of community-based initiatives such as Khululeka.[23] However, it would seem that these new masculinities and identities are very much in the making and these men often end up drawing on more established and hegemonic ideas about masculinity. Khululeka members are also acutely aware that problematic male behaviour such as alcohol abuse remains a serious challenge for some of their members. In

[22] Treatment literacy practitioners were trained by the Treatment Action Campaign (TAC) and MSF to provide HIV/AIDS prevention and treatment knowledge to its members and to the broader community.

[23] MSF, TAC and Khululeka all subscribe to this 'governance from below' approach, yet they are also quite different in their social composition and orientation. MSF is a global NGO of health professionals, TAC a national organisation led largely by professionals with popular participation mostly by unemployed black African women, and Khululeka is a grassroots Community-Based Organisation (CBO) of unemployed and working-class Xhosa men led by someone with tertiary education and employment. Notwithstanding these differences, all three organisations have been involved in common AIDS activist projects and approaches that have created the conditions for the emergence of new social identities, including the new masculinities that seem to be emerging as a result of community-based initiatives such as Khululeka.

other words, these ideas about sexuality and masculinity are still very much in the process of being fleshed out and negotiated.

During a group discussion with Khululeka members in Gugulethu on 18 February 2006, 'Thabo', a forty-something-year-old former ANC liberation fighter, described how diagnosis with AIDS could destroy one's sense of manhood and hope for the future. He recalled that after his diagnosis he had had virtually no support, 'Even my brothers wouldn't support me.' Thabo explained how illness, AIDS stigma, and the fear of dying were a devastating concoction, especially for African men whose identity was intimately tied to sexuality and reproduction. So while Khululeka members were self-consciously seeking to fashion new masculinities they were constrained by their ambivalence and tacit acceptance of dominant conceptions of what it means to be a 'real African man':

> Especially here in Africa, sexual issues are men's pride. Here as an African man you are being judged according to how many women you have. I mean especially among young ones, it's very rare that you find a young man having one girlfriend, for example. Most of the time … men marry more than one wife … Every man judges his future and well being according to the size of his family [laughter from others in the room]. So the doctor says, 'My friend, I'm very sorry you're HIV-positive.' So you just have to stop everything. Imagine that. This makes a vacuum in somebody's heart [laughter]. All the plans you have are gone. So you find out you are HIV-positive and you say, 'I am no longer a man, I have to do away with all my girlfriends.' So this is when the fear and stigma starts. Many people believe that if you're HIV-positive you only have a period of 3 or 5 years and then you're gone [laughter]. And you had all these plans.

Apart from material needs for employment and livelihoods, the need for dignity and respect as a man was a key reason given by members for why Khululeka was established. The need for a safe space for men to address specifically male issues was also put forward as the reason for Khululeka's existence. However, as was mentioned earlier, members also tacitly acknowledged that men, including themselves, remained caught within the discursive webs of dominant masculinities. There seemed to be considerable ambivalence when it came to squaring up to these hegemonic masculinities. This seemed, at times, to be an unwitting confirmation of their endorsement of these hegemonic African masculinities, even as they were seeking to construct new alternatives. The following quotes from participants who attended at a Khululeka workshop at Gordon's Bay, Cape Town, in December 2005 reveal both critical reflexivity and ambivalence as to what it means to be an African man. Many of the statements were also ambiguous as to whether they were referring to 'other men' or to the participants themselves:

> Men often expect to have sex without a condom because they have 'paid' for their wives through *lobola* [bridewealth].
>
> Some men want to sleep around to feel stronger.
>
> I often ask 'Where are the guys in support groups and treatment literacy meetings?' I ask women where their partners are. Many say that they have left them.
>
> Domestic violence is done by us … We are trying to change.
>
> For me, it is very strange to tell my sexual issues to a woman.
>
> Men don't come out openly [about their status]. They are not like women, they are usually

scared. This is the purpose of a men's support group. We talk together about things we can't discuss with female partners.

Most men think that having sex with women is a necessity, but sexual activity generally decreases after diagnosis.

Black men have been oppressed – they lack jobs, housing, shelter, which leads to a higher risk of encountering other social ills such as prostitution … This is not a colour question. It is about poverty and traditions.

Concerns about how to be a responsible father also featured prominently in my discussions with Phumzile. He spoke about how, following his diagnosis, he had suicidal thoughts, 'But then I thought about my children, and what it would be like for them to grow up without a father.' He claimed that even though he had separated from his first wife, his illness had in fact strengthened his relationship with his children. He wanted to provide them with fatherly direction and support. Having got his life back through ARVs, Phumzile was determined to build a future for himself and his family. He remarried an HIV-positive woman and their infant recently tested sero-negative. In 2007 he was employed and his men's support group was growing. Looking back on his life, Phumzile spoke about how he had erred by not taking life, and the threat of HIV, more seriously. He claimed that his lifestyle of sexual recklessness and womanising had led to his HIV-positive status and illness. Given his illness experiences, he was determined to be a responsible father and to teach his children to value life:

I used to take things for granted. I used to ignore things. I used to not to care. I'd say, 'That won't happen to me.' The way I see things now is very much different. That if you don't think of tomorrow, you are nothing. You know, if you don't think of your future, or the people out there, or your kids. That was my major problem. Now I realise my kids wouldn't love to live without their father. Even if I am not staying with them, I must give moral support, give them life, and give them direction to life. So, that's what I'm doing right now. Its time to put my feet on the ground and change the way I see things … At the age of forty you find out that [you] have wasted many years along the way there, doing nothing at all. Not focusing on the right way to succeed. Not having the vision that sometime I could have my own house, my own children, my own car, have a good job, be a father … It's very hard these days, given unemployment and lack of opportunities [but] you have to have a vision.

After Phumzile had returned to good health through ARV treatment he was able to start the long process of remaking his social life, both in terms of his family and personal lifestyle and in relation to his contribution to his community. New conceptions of masculinity, fatherhood, and responsible sexuality were key aspects of this process of identity formation. These notions of 'new life' and 'positive living' influenced his decision to establish Khululeka in 2005.

Conclusion

Calls from South African public health professionals for a new contract between clients and providers, and for the promotion of responsibilised citizenship, resonate with the approach of TAC and MSF. Health professionals and AIDS activists seem to recognise the importance of creating empowered HIV-positive identities and non-hierarchical relations between providers and clients, experts and patients. However, neither of these models of health promotion and rights-based mobilisation adequately acknowledges the problems posed by the deeply embedded character of patriarchal cultures of masculinity. In Chapter 6 it was argued that these rights-based conceptions of a new contract also fail to sufficiently acknowledge the salience of illness experiences in transforming HIV subjectivities and identities. They also fail to recognise the complex mix of religious, communal and activist discourses, interpretations and mediations of these illness and treatment experiences (see Phumzile's testimony in Chapter 6). Yet, it is precisely the discursive power of these interpretive framings of illness and treatment that facilitate the making of new HIV-positive identities and 'responsibilised' subjects, including the kinds of responsible masculinities that Phumzile has sought to create through the formation of Khululeka. Rationalist and liberal individualist conceptions of the modern subject and the rights-bearing citizen are inadequate for understanding the transformative character of these new biosocial processes and identities.

The moral politics of AIDS activism also questions taken-for-granted assumptions about hegemonic masculinities, including the traditional Zulu version performed at Jacob Zuma's rape trial. The Khululeka case suggests that this moral politics can indeed contribute towards innovative community-based attempts to create 'responsibilised masculinities' in a time of AIDS. However, the case study also reveals the precariousness of these innovations, including the ambivalence that Khululeka members themselves express in relation to dominant masculinities. In addition, Khululeka seems to be an isolated community-based initiative in a sea of sexual conservatism and gendered inequalities. It is therefore too early to tell whether such initiatives are indeed capable of challenging hegemonic masculinities. It also remains to be seen whether these initiatives, which are themselves the product of innovative NGO–social movement partnerships, reproduce docile and disciplined subjects of biomedicine and biocapital, or whether they are indeed able to respond to the calls by progressive health professionals and activists for responsible, empowered and knowledgeable patient-citizens.

8
Conclusion
Beyond Rights & the Limits of Liberalism

The case studies in this book have drawn attention to the ambiguous and contradictory character of rights-based approaches to political mobilisation in post-apartheid South Africa. They question assumptions about the individualising and depoliticising nature of rights discourses (Brown 1995). The cases also draw attention to the diverse political rationalities and identities that NGOs and social movements encounter in their daily work. These include hybrid political discourses that defy the enduring binary categories of citizens and subjects, liberals and communitarians, modernists and traditionalists and so on. The NGO and social movement activists discussed in this book appear to have recognised the profoundly hybrid, provisional and situational character of politics in post-apartheid South Africa. The following account of politics in Crossroads, an informal settlement in Cape Town, draws attention to these highly mobile political practices.

In June 1986, during the height of the revolutionary struggle against apartheid, I witnessed the South African Defence Force (SADF) arming Xhosa-speaking vigilantes in a bloody battle against anti-apartheid activists in Crossroads, a shantytown settlement on the outskirts of Cape Town. At the time, I was working with a television crew determined to obtain incriminating footage of security force complicity in fuelling intra-community violence in Crossroads. The SADF and South African Police had clandestinely armed a large group of Xhosa-speaking vigilante elders, referred to in the media either as the *witdoeke*[1] or 'fathers', in an attempt to violently purge Crossroads of militant ANC youth and women's activist organisations that had established strongholds in the informal settlement in the early 1980s.

Deep divisions had emerged in Crossroads as a result of struggles over access to housing, development resources and the presence of ANC youth activists who took control over the People's Courts[2] and enforced consumer boycotts and work

---

[1]   The Afrikaans word *witdoeke* refers to the white head scarves that these 'traditionalists' or 'Fathers' wore during violent confrontations with ANC comrades (*amaqabane*) in Crossroads in 1986.

[2]   These were the forms of popular justice that emerged in many townships in South Africa as a result of the attack on the legitimacy of any apartheid state institutions. The People's Courts sometimes alienated elders by inverting 'traditional' generational hierarchies and delving into the domestic sphere. Many

stayaways. These actions alienated and antagonised many of the elders who participated in the neo-traditional headmen structures (*izibonda*) that existed in the migrant hostels and informal settlements in Cape Town's township. The security forces exploited the tensions between 'fathers' and 'sons' by supporting these conservative elders in their violent battles against anti-apartheid youth activists in Crossroads.

Driving through Crossroads on a misty morning in June 1986 we managed to film police and *witdoeke* collaborating in the torching of hundreds of corrugated iron shacks/homes. We also filmed the charred human remains of 'necklacings' and the dozens of corpses lying alongside the road, the casualties from the previous night's fighting between the machete-wielding *witdoeke* and the ANC comrades (*amaqabane*).

A decade later I spent four days at the Truth and Reconciliation Commission (TRC) hearings into the role of the military in the Crossroads violence. I heard one of the elderly *witdoek* warlords of the 1980s, Sam Ndima, telling Advocate Ndumisa Ntsesebeza, the TRC's head of the investigations unit, that he and his *witdoeke* soldiers were victims of the apartheid state's divide and rule strategies and manipulations. Ndima was now wearing an ANC T-shirt instead of the widely feared *witdoek* he had worn in the 1980s. Ndima spoke about how the youth had usurped power, 'necklacing' alleged *impimpis* (police informers), and undermining traditional authority by setting up youth-controlled People's Courts.

Ndima had managed to reinvent himself as both a victim of apartheid and as a loyal ANC member.[3] He appeared to have created for himself a new political identity to suit the new political times. Clearly, 'traditionalists' such as Ndima were not simply ethnic subjects straitjacketed into tribal identities imposed by the colonial and apartheid regimes (Mamdani 1996). Neither were they the mirror image of the 'western' liberal individualist citizen fighting for his or her rights.

Writing about the persistence of violent patronage politics in Crossroads in the post-apartheid period, Vanessa Watson (2003) draws attention to the conflicting rationalities of modernist planners and the Crossroads leadership and their supporters. She argues that conventional understandings of 'multicultural planning' – as a rational and consensus-building process that encourages cultural tolerance and the accommodation of difference – cannot account for the politics of 'deep difference' which, she argues, explain the continuing violence and political culture of patrimonialism in Crossroads. Whereas planners and city officials envisage 'proper' and 'responsible' citizens who arrive at rational planning solutions through consultation and consensual politics, Watson concludes that the realities on the

---

2 ctnd male elders were publicly flogged as a result of allegations of domestic violence and this contributed towards a backlash against these community policing and popular justice initiatives.

3 Xhosa traditionalists of the 1980s such as Ndima managed to reinvent themselves as loyal members of an African nationalist organisation that had once labelled traditional leadership as an outmoded, anti-modern, antidemocratic and sexist institution whose incumbents had collaborated with the colonial and apartheid authorities. These dramatic shifts in political identity and allegiance became increasingly common as South Africa settled into its new democracy. Former enemies, including members of the Afrikaner National Party joined the ANC and traditional leaders who had participated in the Bantustan system became card-carrying members of the organisation that they had fought and denounced during the apartheid years.

ground suggest that alternative and significantly different political rationalities and subjectivities exist in places like Crossroads. These appear to be inherently incompatible with liberal democratic conceptions of citizenship, rights and civic participation. Watson's analysis of conflict in Crossroads in the post-apartheid period implies that there is an insurmountable impasse between liberal and illiberal political rationalities. But how deep is this 'deep difference'?

It appears that patrimonial and authoritarian styles of politics continue to shape popular struggles over access to low-income housing in informal settlements in Cape Town. This is borne out in the case study of the South African Homeless People's Federation (SAHPF) branch in Victoria Mxenge settlement in Phillipi township (Chapter 4). As a People's Dialogue (PD) NGO activist put it to me, the women in leadership positions at Victoria Mxenge Federation behaved in ways that were identical to the neo-traditional and authoritarian *witdoeke* in Crossroads a decade earlier. But these are not timeless neo-traditionalist political discourses. Instead, they are reproduced under conditions that include deep poverty, unemployment and the virtual collapse of the homelands-based migrant labour economy. The vast majority of urban and rural poor are more or less permanently excluded from active participation in this new democracy and globally connected service economy.

It would appear, though, that political and economic structures that existed during the apartheid period persist in ways that reproduce the kinds of political rationalities and neo-traditional patrimonial politics that Watson writes about. For instance, there is still a shortage of 250,000 houses in Cape Town. This massive shortage of housing for black Africans is itself a legacy of apartheid's homelands and Coloured Labour Preference Area policies. Similarly, economic structures of underdevelopment and chronic poverty in the former homelands of the Eastern Cape Province continue to drive tens of thousands of rural Xhosa-speakers to Cape Town each year. These economic refugees arrive in Cape Town in the search for jobs and better schools, health care services and housing. These historical structures of racialised poverty and underdevelopment reproduce the conditions within which warlordism, patrimonialism, and gangsterism thrive in informal settlements and townships. To get onto a housing list may still require becoming a client of a local warlord or neo-traditional powerbroker.

My brief account of Sam Ndima's appearance before the TRC draws attention to an observation that runs through most of the case studies in this book: that successful interventions by the state, NGOs and social movements require a fine appreciation that political rationalities and identities tend to be deployed situationally. In the 1980s Ndima and his neo-traditional lieutenants had aligned themselves with the apartheid security forces in a violent campaign to reassert traditional authority. By 1996 Ndima had changed his tactics, allegiances and political identity. Ndima's wearing of an ANC T-shirt at the TRC hearings in the mid-1990s suggested that he had switched his political affiliation. He now identified himself with a modern, liberal democratic political organisation that was busy reassessing the place of traditional leaders within a modern Constitutional democracy. Switching sides was a relatively seamless process for Ndima and his lieutenants. They were clearly not trapped within neo-traditional political identities and rationalities.

Instead, there were capable of switching registers, repertoires and identities depending on specific contexts, audiences and political objectives.

How had this transformation taken place, and how did the ANC create the conditions for 'ethnic subjects' like Ndima to so seamlessly morph into new citizens of post-apartheid South Africa? What did the wearing of ANC T-shirts actually signify in terms of the political rationalities of neo-traditionalists such as Ndima?

During the apartheid period the state's homeland (Bantustan) system had sought to straitjacket black South Africans into discrete ethnic categories, subjectivities and territorial units. This massive social engineering project went to enormous lengths to constitute ethnic subjects by buttressing traditional authorities and spending billions of rands creating so-called independent ethnic nation-states scattered throughout South Africa. These separate development policies were also implemented in the cities. For instance, Crossroads violence, much like the violent conflicts between ANC supporters and Inkatha, Gatsha Buthelezi's Zulu cultural national organisation, was a manifestation of state-orchestrated attempts to establish quasi-tribal authorities and tribal enclaves in the heart of South Africa's cities (Robins 1998). These attempts to re-tribalise rural and urban Africans were resisted by anti-apartheid activists and ordinary black South Africans who dismissed Inkatha, Bantustan leaders and traditional authorities as anti-democratic, anti-modern and reactionary apartheid collaborators.

After April 1994, when the ANC government swept into power in the first democratic elections, the former homelands were incorporated into a non-racial, unitary South Africa, and a significant number of the former Bantustan leaders crossed the floor and became ANC MPs in the national and provisional legislatures. Contralesa, the Congress of Traditional Leaders, was also able to win many concessions from the ANC government, and its leader, the shrewd traditional leader and lawyer *Inkosi* Pathekile Holomisa, became an influential ANC Member of Parliament. Revolutionary rhetoric about the overthrow of reactionary chiefs was quickly replaced with official praise poems about chiefs as custodians of tradition. For instance, in 2004 President Mbeki and former president Mandela praised the late paramount chief Kaiser Matanzima, a former Chief Minister of the Transkei homeland, at a funeral in which this former 'Bantustan collaborator' and 'enemy of the people' was eulogised by the ANC leadership as a 'man of the people'. This rehabilitation of former Bantustan leaders and traditional authorities necessitated reconciling patriarchal traditional leadership structures with a rights-based constitution that insisted on gender equality. During the revolutionary struggle the chiefs were seen as simply stooges of the apartheid regime; after apartheid their roles had somehow to be reconciled within a liberal democratic constitutional framework that insisted upon the creation of autonomous rights-bearing citizens rather than ethnic subjects under traditional authorities.

NGOs and social movements became key brokers of this post-apartheid paradigm shift from revolution to liberal democracy, rights and reconciliation. However, this state and civil society-driven project of inculcating liberal conceptions of rights and citizenship was not entirely foreign. These discourses were, to some degree, also part of the anti-apartheid political lexicon of the 1980s. However, the political language of the 1980s did not valorise the virtues of autonomous rights-bearing subjects. Neither did it emphasise the responsibility or accountability of citizens to an illegitimate state. One of the militant slogans of the mass democratic movement was the call to render the townships ungovernable and create liberated zones.

The dramatic transition to democracy in 1994 forced the ANC to transform itself from a revolutionary liberation movement to a responsible, liberal democratic political party and government. This required rendering the townships, and the rest of the country, governable. The ANC's former freedom fighters, now seated in government offices in Pretoria, found themselves facing the enormous task of bringing political and institutional stability to a country that had been virtually brought to its knees by the revolutionary struggle. Non-governmental workers, professionals, workers and students who had identified with the ANC-aligned United Democratic Front (UDF) also struggled to adapt to this dramatically transformed political landscape. Many joined government departments and the NGO sector and became involved in the delivery of housing, water, electricity, development and social and health services.

As the chapters in this book have shown, many post-apartheid NGOs and social movements have become quite adept at mobilising rights in popular struggles to leverage access to state resources. Rights-based approaches have not necessarily translated into the forms of depoliticisation and individualisation assumed by many of liberalism's critics, and neither has 'rights talk' been rendered completely incompatible with group-based claims to 'ethnic' belonging and indigenous identity. The NGO-social movement partnerships discussed in the book developed pragmatic solutions to resolve these political dilemmas. This pragmatism also required recognition of liberalism's limits.

State interventions such as housing provision and employment equity programmes have sought exapnd the black middle class and provide resources to the black working class and the poor. The delivery of housing, land, health and social services has also been about pedagogies of liberal citizenship and governmentality (Robins 2002). However, from the perspective of the NGOs and social movements discussed in this book, rights, citizenship and state programmes are clearly not the only games in town. These organisations also recognised that to realise rights required the mass mobilisation of poor communities through the creation of solidarities and 'social capital'. The case studies in this book analysed the complex, contradictory and ambiguous roles of NGO workers and activists as brokers and mediators of 'rights talk' as well as agents of mass mobilisation in poor communities.

During the 1980s, the ANC, UDF, trade union movement and civic organisations were seen as the vanguard of the liberation struggle in South Africa. These organisations were involved in mass mobilisation that produced highly effective outcomes. The post-apartheid period witnessed the emergence of new social movements (NSMs) addressing a wide range of issues that went well beyond the narrowly political concerns of the 1970s and 1980s. The Treatment Action Campaign (TAC), the South African Homeless People's Federation (SAHPF) and the San and Nama indigenous people's movements are examples of globally connected NGO–social movement partnerships that seek to use rights talk and collective mobilisation to ensure that the poor and excluded gain access to the fruits of democracy and development.

These pragmatic reformist strategies differ markedly from those of the more radical and millenarian politics of anti-globalisation movements. They also differ from the identity-based new social movements of the North that critics such as Marc Edelman (2001) and Wendy Brown (1995) regard as being responsible for promoting individualisation, fragmentation and depoliticisation, and thereby undermining the possibility of an emancipatory politics that could seriously challenge the global hegemony of neoliberal capitalism. The case studies in this book show how these NGO–social movement partnerships strategically and situationally deploy the language and practices of liberal democracy, while not necessarily buying into the tenets and ideology of (neo)liberal capitalism. TAC's legal challenge to the global pharmaceutical industry over drug patents is an excellent case in point (see Chapter 5).

The case studies also draw attention to the limited capacity of liberal states, NGOs and social movements to completely capture the hearts and minds of the target populations of their projects and programmes. Citizens can, like Gören Hyden's 'uncaptured peasantry'(1980), circumvent, elude, reconfigure or resist state and civil society programmes and political discourses. For the chronically poor and unemployed, fully participating in formal political and economic worlds may limit future prospects and possibilities. In response, the urban and rural poor are often obliged to adopt highly opportunistic, mobile, provisional and improvisational forms of engagement with government, donor and NGO programmes. For example, they may straddle multiple nodes of belonging and affiliation that could include participation in liberal democratic programmes of nation-building, rights and citizenship alongside membership of global social movements and/or neighbourhood gangs, anti-crime vigilante groups, religious movements and neo-traditional authority structures.

This multiplicity of shifting affiliations and identities can challenge attempts to inculcate pedagogies of liberal citizenship that envisage the classical autonomous rights-bearing citizens detached from parochial ties of kinship, neighbourhood and ethnic clan. The cases suggest that for the chronically poor, the more affiliations and networks the better. Citizens may therefore not be so seamlessly captured by state discourses as some Foucaultian analysts of the surveillance state seem to suggest. These opportunistic strategies, which are of course not exclusive to the poor and those living in the Third World, can become well suited to conditions of extreme uncertainty and instability. The NGO–social movement partnerships discussed in this book have had to address and accommodate these conditions of radical contingency that impact upon the lives of the people they work with. So how are NGOs and social movements to mobilise their constituencies given these conditions of radical contingency and uncertainty?

It was mentioned in Chapter 4 that during the anti-apartheid period there was a palpable sense of community solidarity and heroic revolutionary resistance by militant youth activists in the townships. The political language of revolutionary struggle was then not about rights but was rather concerned with radical transformation of the economy and society. The Mass Democratic Movement (MDM) drew together working-class communities, trade unions, churches, mosques, black and white middle-class professionals, university students, and other sectors of South African society that shared this vision of transformation. The United Democratic Front (UDF) was the public face of this non-racial, multi-class political movement. With the demise of apartheid, the UDF folded into ANC party structures. The new government soon came to view militant community-based mobilisation, revolutionary politics and mass protest as unruly, and as constituting a threat to law and order. Mass mobilisation after apartheid was no longer encouraged by the ANC revolutionaries-turned-bureaucrats. The militant 'Young Lions' of the 1980s who were unable to find their place in this new South Africa tended to be pathologised and labelled as the 'Lost Generation.'

There was also a tendency for ANC officials to discredit militant community mobilisation against privatisation policies, housing evictions, the failure of government delivery, and the introduction of cost-recovery measures for water, electricity and other services. Terms such as the 'ultra-Left' were used by government officials to label and discredit leaders of social movements such as COSATU, TAC, SECC, and the Anti-Evictions Campaign. The organisations discussed in this book did not warrant the label 'ultra-Left'. They adopted rights-based approaches that seemed to reflect a commitment to liberal democracy while at the same recognising the limits of liberalism. These organisations were not stooges of neo-liberal capital and slaves to rights talk, but neither were they exemplars of revolutionary movements.

The cases also revealed the ways in which activists' rights-based approaches at times clashed with authoritarian and anti-democratic forms of local politics and governance (see Chapters 4 and 5). For instance, AIDS activists had to address local responses of intolerance, denial, stigma and sexual violence, for instance the cases of AIDS activists Gugu Dlamini and Lorna Mlofana, both of whom were killed by community members after revealing their HIV-positive status. Clearly, lofty liberal ideals of rights, citizenship, civil society and 'deep democracy' needed to be tempered by the recognition of the authoritarian, patriarchal and gendered forms of violence that occurred in many of the places in which NGOs and social movements operated. These everyday realities also pose serious policy dilemmas for liberal democracy in South Africa. For example, how does the liberal state reconcile gender equality provisions in the Constitution with patriarchal traditional leadership structures and everyday practices of violence against women? These contradictions, which are themselves products of colonial and apartheid legacies of violence and inequalities, present major challenges to civil society organisations seeking to promote the ideas and practices of liberal democracy, rights and citizenship.

The case studies suggest that these challenges cannot always be met using conventional state and NGO-driven programmes and pedagogies of citizenship. Instead, we need to begin to better understand the social, existential and religious experiences and meaning-making processes of citizens such as the AIDS activists referred to in Chapter 6. These activist accounts of the passage from 'near death' to 'new life' provide insights into how ordinary people make sense of their lives and experiences of social suffering and exclusion. These accounts also hint at how NGO and social movement activists could begin to recollect and recast the fading memories and practices of the liberation struggle as they proceed to transform today's rhetoric of rights and citizenship into realisable goals and progressive, emancipatory projects.

This pragmatic politics of critical engagement with the state and democratic discourses also has to take cognisance of the structural limits of South Africa's liberal democracy – massive unemployment, chronic poverty, everyday violence, racial and class inequality (racial capitalism), the AIDS pandemic and so on (see Terreblanche 2002). The Crossroads neo-traditionalist vigilante-turned-loyal ANC member, the former revolutionary-turned-billionaire, the Bantustan traditional leader-turned ANC loyalist, and the former National Party apparatchik-turned-ANC MP, all appear to have reinvented themselves in the new South Africa. Similarly, NGOs and social movements have had to make a radical paradigm shift from revolution to rights talk. For the NGO-social movement partnerships discussed in this book, rights-based modes of mobilisation appear to have been reasonably effective ways of pushing at the limits of liberalism.

The book has argued that the complexity of social and political life on the margins forces us to rethink the three propositions discussed in the Introduction. The case studies offered an alternative perspective on the politics of rights and collective action in post-apartheid South Africa by highlighting the ambiguous and contradictory character of rights-based approaches to political mobilisation. They also questioned taken-for-granted assumptions about the individualising, fragmenting and depoliticising nature of rights discourses. This challenges some of the more cynical analyses suggesting an 'end of politics' referred to in the discussion of 'Proposition 1'. By arguing for the continued salience of NGOs, social movements and other civil society actors in creating new forms of democratic citizenship, collective action, political subjectivity and identity, the case studies interrogated the sanitised prescriptions of 'good governance' that are so often touted by donors and development agencies. Instead they suggest the need for the recognition of the complex, hybrid and ambiguous relationships between civil society and the state that involve new negotiations around citizenship, identity and political subjectivity which emerge in particular contexts.

The cases also interrogate 'Proposition 2' by drawing attention to the diverse political rationalities and identities that NGO and social movements encounter in their daily work. These include hybrid political discourses that defy the enduring binary categories of citizens and subjects, liberals and communitarians, modernists and traditionalists and so on (see Proposition 2). The case studies of NGO and social movement partnerships suggest that NGOs and community activists have indeed taken cognisance of the profoundly hybrid, provisional and situational character of politics in marginalised communities in South Africa. These examples of NGO and social movement strategic partnerships offer donors, development agencies, the state and the broader civil society sector, models for engaging with this complex politics of the margins. They can also contribute towards providing more nuanced understandings of the shifting relationships between the state, civil society and the popular classes (Proposition 3).

Not all of the cases discussed in the book were equally successful. For instance, the indigenous rights movement that emerged in the Northern Cape Province had limited success in terms of uplifting its members economically. While it was successful in its land claims, in gaining media attention for its campaigns, and in forging linkages with global indigenous rights movements and donors, the majority of its rank-and-file members remained stuck in chronic poverty and unemployment in the semi-arid Northern Cape Province, one of the most underdeveloped regions in South Africa.

In the case of SAHPF, the movement established strong linkages with other SDI affiliates, and hundreds of low-income houses were built by VMx federation members with SAHPF loans. However, the case study of the Cape Town federation leadership draws attention to the divergence between the SAHPF and SDI's ideology of horizontal, non-hierarchical and decentralised leadership, and the political culture of patronage, hierarchy and centralised leadership that was deeply embedded in Cape Town's urban townships.

When it came to TAC, the AIDS movement had successes on a number of fronts. Its successes could be attributed to the following factors: savvy media campaigns, strategic litigation combined with grassroots mobilisation, strong and charismatic leadership, powerful moral arguments, which together with litigation, convinced the state and the global pharmaceutical industry to make anti-retroviral therapy available to poor people. The success of TAC has also been due to its ability to sustain itself beyond a single campaign, that is, the struggle for the provision of ARVs in the public health system. TAC has also been able to create and support new initiatives and offshoots such as the support group for men living with HIV (see Chapter 7).

What these movements and their offshoots share is a recognition that they need to develop hybrid and situated strategies to leverage the state in order to access resources, i.e. strategies that deploy rights talk and communitarian logics of collective mobilisation. This has contributed towards a pragmatic politics that differs markedly from the more militant and ideologically-driven anti-globalisation movements such as the Anti-Eviction Campaign, the Anti-Privatisation Forum, the Soweto Electricity Crisis Committee and the Landless Peoples Movement. In addition, the indigenous rights movement and TAC seemed to have been extraordinarily successful in soliciting public interest in their campaigns through a strategic combination of litigation and savvy media strategies. Along with the SAHPF case, the indigenous rights and AIDS activist causes were also viewed favourably by donors and the state, not withstanding ongoing conflicts between AIDS activists and the national Health Minister.

By contrast, the anti-globalisation movement in South Africa has tended to get involved in direct confrontation with the state and global capital. It is therefore perhaps not surprising that organisations such as the Landless Peoples Movement and the Anti-Privatisation Forum have been labelled as belonging to the 'unpatriotic ultra-Left' by senior ANC government officials concerned with possible disruption that such movements may pose to the economy and national security. These organisations have also been the target of state intelligence surveillance, suggesting that the state is indeed concerned about the threat they may pose.

They have also failed to gain much public response and media visibility, perhaps because their concerns with housing, land and macro-economic policy do not generate the same sense of immediacy as the AIDS pandemic. These more militant movements have, however, highlighted the serious problems of structural unemployment and the failings of state service delivery and social transformation. These anti-globalisation movements have not, however, had anything like the successes of the trade union movement in terms of campaigns and social mobilisation.

There were of course many omissions in terms of the scope of this book. For instance, the book did not focus on national organisations such as COSATU, one of the most politically influential and largest social movements in South Africa. Notwithstanding its political strength, COSATU is facing serious problems as global capital and economic liberalisation wreak havoc with domestic manufacturing industries. In addition, the South African economy is increasingly shifting towards a service economy concentrating on information technology (IT), financial services and tourism sectors. Yet, in March 2007, COSATU leader Zwelinzima Vavi returned from meetings with trade unionists and Left leaders in South America convinced that the time had come for the popular Left to drive out the 'neo-liberal elements' from the ANC (*Mail & Guardian*, 9 March 2007, p. 4). Given COSATU's backing for former deputy President Jacob Zuma (see Chapter 7), as well as the groundswell of popular support that emrged for both the popular Left and Zuma in the run-up to the presidential succession race, it is not inconceivable that the ANC could give way to this concerted push from the Left. In the shadow of these looming national political showdowns, however, are the innovative and remarkably successful NGO-social movement collaborations that have been discussed in this book. It is here, in the political margins, that new, improvised and hybrid forms of mobilisation, citizenship and political identities are emerging.

Bibliography

Adams, V. and Pigg, S.L. (eds) 2005. *Sex in Development: Science, Sexuality, and Morality in Global Perspective*. Durham, NC and London: Duke University Press.

Agamben, G. 1998. *Homo Sacer*. (Translated by Daniel Heller-Roazen). Stanford, CA: Stanford University Press.

Alvarez, S.E. 1998. 'Latin American Feminisms "Go Global": Trends of the 1990s and Challenges for the New Millennium', in Alvarez, S., Dagnino, E. and Escobar, A. (eds) *Culture of Politics/Politics of Cultures: Re-visioning Latin American Social Movements*. Boulder, CO: Westview Press: pp. 293–324.

Alvarez, S.E., Dagnino E. and Escobar, A. (eds) 1998. *Culture of Politics, Politics of Cultures: Re-visioning Latin American Social Movements*. Boulder, CO: Westview Press.

Appadurai, A. 2001. *Globalization*. Durham, NC: Duke University Press.

— 2002a. 'Grassroots Globalization and the Research Imagination', in Vincent, J. (ed.) *The Anthropology of Politics: A Reader in Ethnography, Theory and Critique*. Malden, MA: Blackwell.

— 2002b. 'Deep Democracy: Urban Governmentality and the Horizon of Politics', *Public Culture*, 14(1): 21–47.

Appadurai, A. and Holston, J. 1999. 'Cities and Citizenship', *Public Culture* (8)2: 187–204.

Appiah, K. 1992. *In My Father's House: Africa in the Philosophy of Culture*. Oxford: Oxford University Press.

Arendt, H. 1958. *The Human Condition*. Chicago: University of Chicago Press.

Armstrong, D. 1995. 'The Rise of Surveillance Medicine', *Sociology of Health and Illness*, 17: 393–404.

Barry, A., Osborne, T. and Rose, N. (eds) 1996. *Foucault and Practical Reason: Liberalism, Neo-Liberalism and Rationalities of Government*. London: University College London Press.

Bauman, Z. 1999. *In Search of Politics*. London: Polity Press.

— 2001. *Community: Seeking Safety in an Insecure World*. London: Polity Press.

Bauman, Ted. 2006. 'Utshani Fund and the SAHPF in Cape Town', *The Facts* newsletter, May: 2.

Bayart, J-F. 1993. *The State in Africa: Politics of the Belly*. New York: Longman.

Bayart, J-F., Ellis, S. and Hibou, B. (eds) 1999. *The Criminalisation of the State in Africa*. Bloomington: Indiana University Press; Oxford: James Currey in association with the International African Institute.

Beck, U. 1992. *Risk Society: Towards a New Modernity*. New Delhi: Sage.

Benatar, S. 2004. 'Health Policy Report: Health Care Reform and the Crisis of HIV and AIDS in South Africa', *The New England Journal of Medicine* 351(1): 81–92; www.nejm.org

Bhabha, H. 1990. *Location of Culture*. London and New York: Routledge.

Biehl, J. 2001. 'Vita: Life in a Zone of Social Abandonment', *Social Text* 19(3): 131–49.

— 2004. 'The Activist State: Global Pharmaceuticals, AIDS and Citizenship in Brazil', *Social Text* 22(3): 105–32.

— 2005. *Vita: Life in a Zone of Social Abandonment*. Berkeley: Los Angeles and London: University of California Press.

Bond, P. 2000. *Elite Transition: From Apartheid to Neoliberalism in South Africa*. London: Pluto Press.

Boonzaier, E. 1987. 'From Communal Grazing to "Economic Units": Changing Access to Land in a Namaqualand Reserve', *Development South Africa*, 4(3): 479–91.

— 1996. 'Negotiating the Development of Tourism in the Richtersveld, South Africa', in Price, M. (ed.) *People and Tourism in Fragile Environments*. Chichester, UK: John Wiley and Sons, pp. 123–37.

Boonzaier, E. and Sharp, J. (eds) 1998. *South African Keywords: The Uses and Abuses of Political Concepts*. Cape Town: David Philip Press.

— 1993. 'Staging Ethnicity: Lessons from Namaqualand', *Track Two*, February 1993: 10–13.

— 1994. 'Ethnic Identity and Performance: Lessons from Namaqualand', *Journal of Southern African Studies,* 20(3): 405–15.

Brown, W. 1995. *States of Injury: Power and Freedom in Late Modernity*. Princeton, NJ: Princeton University Press.

Caldwell, J.C., Caldwell, P., and Orubuloye, I.O. 1992. 'The Family and Sexual Networking in Sub-Saharan Africa: Historical and Regional Differences and Present Day Implications', *Population Studies* 46(3): 385–410.

Cameron, E. 2005. *Witness to AIDS*. Cape Town: Tafelberg.

Castro Hlongwane, Caravans, Cats, Geese, Foot and Mouth and Statistics: HIV/AIDS and the Struggle for the Humanisation of the Africans, anonymous text posted on the ANC website on March 2002.

Channock, M. 1985. *Law, Custom, and Social Order: The Colonial Experience in Malawi and Zambia*. Portsmouth, NH: Heinemann.

Chatterjee, P. 1993. *The Nation and Its Fragments: Colonial and Postcolonial Histories*. Princeton, NJ: Princeton University Press.

— 2004. *The Politics of the Governed: Reflections on Popular Politics in Most of the World*. New York: Columbia University Press.

Clifford, J. 1988. *The Predicament of Culture: Twentieth-Century Ethnography, Literature and Art*. Cambridge, MA, and London: Harvard University Press.

Coetzee, D. and Schneider, H. 2004. 'Editorial', *South African Medical Journal* 93(10): 1–3.

Coetzee, J.M. 1999. *Disgrace*. London: Secker and Warburg.

Cohen, R. and Rai, S.M. (eds) 2000a. 'Introduction', *in Global Social Movements*. Brunswick, NJ and London: Athlone Press, pp. 1–17.

— 2000b. *Global Social Movements*. New Brunswick, NJ and London: Athlone Press.

Cole, J. 1987. *The Politics of Reform and Repression 1976–1986*. Cape Town: David Philip.

Comaroff, J. 2002. 'Governmentality, Materiality, Legality, Modernity: On the Colonial State in Africa', in Deutsch, J-G., P. Probst and H. Schmidt (eds) *African Modernities*. Oxford: James Currey; Portsmouth, NJ: Heinemann.

— n.d. 'Beyond the Politics of Bare Life: AIDS and the Neoliberal Order'. A paper presented at the Berlin symposium on 'AIDS and the Moral Order', March 3–6, 2005, Berlin.

Comaroff, J.L. and Comaroff, J. (eds) 1999. *Civil Society and the Political Imagination in Africa: Critical Perspectives*. Chicago and London: Chicago University Press.

— 2005. 'Reflections on Liberalism, Policulturalism and ID–ology', in Robins, S. (ed.) *Limits to Liberation after Apartheid: Citizenship, Governance and Culture*. Oxford: James Currey.

— (forthcoming) *Ethnicity Inc.*

Connell, R.W. 1996. *Masculinities*. Berkeley: University of California Press.

Cooper, F. and Packard, R.M. (eds) 1997. *International Development and the Social Sciences: Essays on the History and Politics of Knowledge*. Berkeley, Los Angeles, London: University of California Press.

Cornwall, A. and Lindisfarne, N. 1994. 'Dislocating Masculinity: Gender, Power and Anthropology', in Cornwall, A. and Lindisfarne, N. (eds) *Dislocating Masculinity: Comparative Ethnographies*. London: Routledge: pp. 11–47.

Cowan, J.K., Dembour, M. and Wilson, R.A. (eds) 2001. *Culture and Rights: Anthropological Perspectives*. Cambridge: Cambridge University Press.

Crush, J. (ed.) 1995. *Power of Development*. London and New York: Routledge.

Das, V. and Poole, D. (eds) 2004. *Anthropology in the Margins of the State*. Sante Fe: School of American Research Press; Oxford: James Currey.

Davis, M. 1990. *City of Quartz: Excavating the Future of Los Angeles*. London: Verso.

Deacon, B., Hulse, M. and Stubbs, P. 1997. *Global Social Policy: International Organizations and the Future of Welfare*. London: Sage.

Delius, P. and Glaser, C. 2002. 'Sexual Socialisation in South Africa: A Historical Perspective', *African Studies*, 61(1): 27–54.

Denzin, N. K. 1987. *The Recovering Alcoholic*. London and New Delhi: Sage.

Department of Health, 2003. Report: Men in HIV/AIDS Partnerships: Provincial Consultative Workshops (May–July 2003): 'Men care enough to act'. Pretoria: Department of Health.

Deutsch, J–G., Probst, P. and Schmidt, H. (eds) 2002. *Perspectives on African Modernities*. Oxford: James Currey.

Dorrington, R., Bourne D., Bradshaw D., Laubscher, R. and Timaeus, I. 2001. *The Impact of HIV/AIDS on Adult Mortality in South Africa* (Medical Research Council Technical Report, Burden of Disease Research Unit (MRC)).

Edelman, M. 2001. 'Social Movements: Changing Paradigms and Forms of Politics', *Annual Review of Anthropology*, 30: 285–317.

Epstein, S. 1996. *Impure Science: AIDS, Activism and the Politics of Knowledge*. Berkeley: University of California Press.

Erlmann, V. 1992. 'The Past is Far and the Future is Far: Power and Performance Among Zulu Migrant Workers', *American Ethnologist*, 19(4): 688–709.

Escobar, A. 1995. *Encountering Development: The Making and Unmaking of the Third World*. Princeton, NJ: Princeton University Press.

Escobar, A. and Alvarez, S.E. (eds). 1992. *The Making of Social Movements in Latin America: Identity Strategy and Democracy*. Boulder, CO: Westview Press.

Esteva, G. 1992. 'Development, in Sachs, W. (ed.) *The Development Dictionary: A Guide to Knowledge and Power*. London: Zed Books.

Falk, R. 1993. 'The Making of Global Citizenship', in Childs, J.B., Brecher, J. and Cutler, J. (eds) *Global Visions: Beyond the New World Order*. Boston, MA: South End, pp. 39–50.

Farmer, P. 1992. *AIDS and Accusation: Haiti and the Geography of Blame*. Berkeley and Los Angeles: University of California Press.

— 2004. 'An Anthropology of Structural Violence', *Current Anthropology*, 45(3): 305.

Fassin, E. 2006. 'The Rise and Fall of Sexual Politics in the Public Sphere: A Transatlantic Contrast', *Public Culture*, 18(1): 79–110.

Ferguson, J. 1990. *The Anti-Politics Machine: 'Development', Depoliticization and Bureaucratic State Power in Lesotho*. Cambridge: Cambridge University Press.

— 1999. *Expectations of Modernity: Myths and Meanings of Urban Life on the Zambian Copperbelt*. Berkeley: University of California Press.

Fisher, W. 1997. '"Doing Good": The Politics and Antipolitics of NGO Practices', *Annual Review of Anthropology* 26: 439–64.

Friedman, S. and Mottiar, S. 2004. 'Rewarding Engagements? The Treatment Action Campaign and the Politics of HIV/AIDS'. Joint project between Centre of Civil Society and School of Development Studies, University of KwaZulu–Natal.

Friends of Jacob Zuma Website. http: //www.friendsofjz.co.za/viewmessage.asp.

Fukuyama, F. 1992. *The End of History and the Last Man*. New York: Free Press.

Garland, E. 1999. 'Developing Bushmen: Building Civil(ized) Society in the Kalahari and Beyond', in Comaroff, J.L. and Comaroff, J. (eds) *Civil Society and the Political Imagination in Africa: Critical Perspectives*. Chicago: University of Chicago Press.

Gaventa, John. 2002. 'Exploring Citizenship, Participation and Accountability', *IDS Bulletin* 33(2), 1–10.

Geertz, C. 1960. 'The Changing Role of the Cultural Broker', *Comparative Studies in Social History*, 2.

Geschiere, P. and Nyamnjoh, F. 2002. 'Capitalism and Autochthony: The Seesaw of Mobility and Belonging', in John and Jean Comaroff (eds) *Millennial Capitalism and the Culture of Neoliberalism*. Raleigh, NC: Duke University Press.

Giddens, A. 1991. *Modernity and Self-identity: Self and Society in the Late Modern Age*. Cambridge: Polity Press.

Gills, B., Rocamora, J., and Wilson, R. (eds) 1993. *Low-Intensity Democracy: Political Power in the New World Order*. Boulder, CO: Pluto.

Gilroy, P. 1993. *The Black Atlantic: Double Consciousness and Modernity*. Cambridge: Cambridge University Press.

Gitay, J. 2002. 'Rhetoric, Politics, Science, Medicine: The South African HIV/AIDS Controversy'. Unpublished paper, Centre for African Studies, University of Cape Town, 18 September.

Goffman, E. 1971. *Relations in Public.* New York: Harper Colophon Books.

Gordon, E.R. 1992. *The Bushman Myth and the Making of a Namibian Underclass,* Boulder, CO: Westview Press.

Green, J.M. 1999. *Deep Democracy: Community, Diversity and Transformation.* Lanham, MD: Rowan and Littlefield.

Gupta, A. 1998. *Postcolonial Developments: Agriculture in the Making of Modern India.* Durham, NC and London: Duke University Press.

Hamilton, C. 1998. *Terrific Majesty: The Powers of Shaka Zulu and the Limits of Historical Invention.* Cambridge, MA: Harvard University Press.

Hann, C. and Dunn E. (eds) 1996. *Civil Society: Challenging Western Models.* New York: Routledge.

Hardt, M. and Negri, A. 2000. *Empire.* Cambridge, MA: Harvard University Press.

Heald, S. 1995. 'The Power of Sex: Some Reflections on the Caldwells' "African Sexuality" Thesis', *Africa* 65(4): 489–505.

Held, D. (ed.) 1993. *Prospects for Democracy.* London: Polity Press.

Hoad, N., Martin, K. and Reid, G. (eds) 2005. *Sex and Politics in South Africa.* Cape Town: Double Storey.

Hobsbawm, E. and Ranger, T. (eds) 1983. *The Invention of Tradition.* New York: Cambridge University Press.

Holston, J. and Appadurai, A. 1996. 'Cities and Citizenship', *Public Culture* 8: 187–204.

Hunter, Mark. 2006. 'Fathers without *Amandla*: Zulu-speaking Men and Fatherhood', in Richter, L. and Morrell, R. (eds) *Baba: Men and Fatherhood in South Africa.* Cape Town: Human Sciences Research Council Press.

Hunter, Monica. 1979 (1936). *Reaction to Conquest: Effects of Contact with Europeans on the Pondo of South Africa.* Cape Town: David Philip.

— 2005. 'Cultural politics and masculinities: Multiple–partners in historical perspective in Kwa-Zulu Natal', in Reid, G. and Walker, L. (eds) *Men Behaving Differently: South African Men Since 1994.* Cape Town: Double Storey.

— (forthcoming) 'Was the Scale of the South African AIDS Pandemic Inevitable?: Rethinking the Political Economy of Sex in Contemporary South Africa', *Social Science and Medicine.*

Hyden, G. 1980. *Beyond Ujamaa in Tanzania: Underdevelopment and an Uncaptured Peasantry.* Berkeley: University of California Press.

Irwin, A. 1995. *Citizen Science: A Study of People, Expertise and Sustainable Development.* London and New York: Routledge.

James, D. 2000a. 'Hill of Thorns: Custom, Knowledge and the Reclaiming of a Lost Land in the New South Africa', *Development and Change* 31: 629–49.

— 2000b. '"After Years in the Wilderness": The Discourse of Land Claims in the New South Africa', *The Journal of Peasant Studies* 27 (3) 142–61.

Jeannerat, C. 1995. 'Invocations of the Female *Vhusha* Ceremony and the Struggle for Identity and Security in Tshiendeulu, Venda.' Paper presented at the conference of Association of Anthropologists of South Africa, Grahamstown, September 1995.

Jones, E. and Gaventa, J. (eds) 2002. *Concepts of Citizenship: A Review.* Brighton, UK: Institute of Development Studies.

Kamat, S. 2003. 'NGOs and the New Democracy: The False Saviors of International Development', *Harvard International Review,* 25.

— 2005. 'The NGO-ization of Grassroots Politics', in Leistyna, P. (ed.) *Cultural Studies: from Theory to Action.* Oxford: Blackwell.

Kistner, U. 2004. 'Sovereign Power and Bare Life with HIV/AIDS: Bio-Politics South African Style'. Paper presented at the Wits Institute for Social and Economic Research (WISER) conference entitled 'Life and Death in the Time of AIDS', October, http: // wiserweb.wits.ac.za/PDF%20Files/biopolitics%20–%20kirstner.PDF

Koelble, T.A. and LiPuma, E. 2005. 'Traditional Leaders and Democracy: Culture Politics in the Age of Globalisation', in Robins, S. (ed.) *Limits to Liberation after Apartheid: Citizenship, Governance and Culture.* Oxford: James Currey.

Kuper, A. 2003. 'The Return of the Native', *Current Anthropology*, Vol. 44(3).

Latour, B. 1993. *We Have Never Been Modern.* Cambridge, MA: Harvard University Press.

— 2004. 'Why has Critique Run out of Steam? From Matters of Fact to Matters of Concern', *Critical Inquiry* 30: 225–48.

— 2005. 'Why has Critique Run out of Steam? From Matters of Fact to Matters of Concern', http: //www.ensmp.fr/~latour/articles/article/089.html.

Leach, M. 2005. *MMR Mobilization: Citizens and Science in a British Vaccine Controversy.* IDS Working Paper 247. Brighton, UK: Institute of Development Studies.

Leach, M., Scoones, I. and Wynne, B. (eds) 2005. *Science and Citizens: Globalization and the Challenge of Engagement.* London and New York: Zed Books.

Lebert, T. 2004. 'Municipal commonage as a form of land redistribution: A Case Study of the New Forms of Leliefontein, a Communal Reserve in Namaqualand, South Africa'. Research report no. 18. Programme for Land and Agrarian Studies, University of the Western Cape, November.

Leclerc-Madlala, S. 2004. 'Transactional Sex and the Pursuit of Modernity'. Centre for Social Science Research (CSSR) Working Paper No. 68. Cape Town: Centre for Social Science Research, University of Cape Town.

Lee, Richard. 1979. *The !Kung San: Men, Women, and Work in a Foraging Society.* Cambridge, MA: Harvard University Press.

Levi, P. 1979. *If This is a Man – The Truce.* London: Penguin Books.

Lévi-Strauss, C. 1966. *The Savage Mind.* London: Weidenfeld and Nicolson.

Luckham, R. 1998. 'Are There Alternatives to Liberal Democracy?', in Robinson, M. and White, G. (eds) *The Democratic Developmental State. Politics and Institutional Design.* Oxford: Oxford University Press.

Mafeje, A. 1971. 'Ideology of Tribalism', *Journal of Modern African Studies*, 4(2).

Magubane, B. 1973. 'The Xhosa in Town Revisited: Urban Social Anthropology – A Failure in Method and Theory', *American Anthropologist*, 75: 1701–14.

Mail & Guardian, Jacob Zuma Special Report. http: //www.mg.co.za/specialreport. aspx?area=zuma_report

Mamdani, M. 1996. *Citizen and Subject: Contemporary Africa and the Legacy of Late Colonialism.* Princeton, NJ: Princeton University Press; London: James Currey.

Marais, H. 1998. *South Africa: Limits to Change: The Political Economy of Transformation.* London: Zed Books.

Mbembe, A. 2001. *On the Postcolony.* Berkeley and Los Angeles: University of California Press.

Marcus, T. 2001. 'Kissing the Cobra: Sexuality and High Risk in a Generalised Epidemic – a Case Study', paper presented at the conference 'AIDS in Context', University of the Witwatersrand, Johannesburg, March.

Melucci, A. 1989. *Nomads of the Present: Social Movements and Individual Needs in Contemporary Society*. Philadelphia: Temple University Press.

Merry, S. E. 2001. 'Spatial Governmentality and the New Urban Social Order: Controlling Gender Violence Through Law', *American Anthropologist*, 103: 16–29.

Migdal, J. 1988. *Strong Societies and Weak States: State–Society Relations and State Capabilities in the Third World*. Princeton, NJ: Princeton University Press.

Mills, D. and Ssewakiryanga, R. 2005. 'No Romance Without Finance: Commodities, Masculinities and Relationships amongst Kampalan Students', in Cornwell, A. (ed.) *Readings in Gender in Africa*. Oxford: James Currey.

Mitlin, D., L. Podlashuc and J. Bolnick. 2003. IIED Case Study: South African Homeless People's Federation, Cape Town, South Africa. Unpublished People's Dialogue document.

Moffett, H. 2006. '"These Women, They Force Us to Rape Them": Rape as Narrative of Social Control in Post Apartheid South Africa', *Journal of Southern African Studies*, 32(1): 129–49.

Monga, C. 1996. *The Anthropology of Anger: Civil Society and Democracy in Africa*. (Translated by Linda L. Fleck and Celestin Monga). Boulder, CO: Lynne Rienner.

Moodie, D. 1994. *Going For Gold*. Berkeley: University of California Press.

Moore, D. 1993. 'Contesting Terrain in Zimbabwe's Eastern Highlands: Political Ecology and Peasant Resource Struggles'. Paper submitted to *Economic Geography*.

Morrell, R. (ed.) 2001. *Changing Men in South Africa*. London: Zed Books.

Nguyen, V-K. 2005. 'Antiretroviral Globalism, Biopolitics, and Therapeutic Citizenship', in Ong, A. and Collier, S. J. (eds) *Global Assemblages: Technology, Politics, and Ethics as Anthropological Problems*. Oxford: Blackwell.

Niehaus, I. 2002. 'Renegotiating Masculinity in the South African Lowveld: Narratives of Male–Male Sex in Labour Compounds and in Prisons', *African Studies*, 61(1): 77–97.

Niehaus, I. 2005. 'Masculine Domination in Sexual Violence: Interpreting Accounts of Three Cases of Rape in the South African Lowveld', in Reid, G. and Walker, L. (eds) *Men Behaving Differently: South African Men Since 1994*. Cape Town: Double Storey.

Ntsebeza, L. 2005. *Democracy Compromised: Chiefs and the Politics of Land in South Africa*. Leiden: Brill.

Nyamnjoh, F. 2002. '"A Child is One Person's Only in the Womb": Domestication, Agency, and Subjectivity in the Cameroonian Grassfields', in Werbner, R. (ed.) *Postcolonial Subjectivities in Africa*. New York: Zed Books.

Ong, A. 1999. 'Clash of Civilizations or Asian Liberalism? An Anthropology of the State and Citizenship', in Moore, H. (ed.) *Anthropological Theory Today*. Cambridge: Polity Press.

Ouzgane, L. and Morrell, R. (eds) 2005. *African Masculinities: Men in Africa from the Late Nineteenth Century to the Present*. New York: Palgrave Macmillan and Durban: University of Kwa-Zulu Natal Press.

Paine, R. 1971. 'A Theory of Patronage and Brokerage', in Paine, R. (ed.) *Patrons and Brokers in the East Arctic*. St John's: Memorial University. Newfoundland, pp. 8–21.

Paley, J. 2002. 'Toward an Anthropology of Democracy', *Annual Review of Anthropology*, 31: 469–96.

People's Dialogue. 2003. 'uTshani BuyaKhuluma'. Cape Town: PD.

Petras, J. 1997. 'Imperialism and NGOs in Latin America', *Monthly Review*, 49: 10–27.

Petras, J. and Veltmeyer, H. 2001. *Globalisation Unmasked*. London and New York: Zed Press.

Petryna, A. 2002. *Life Exposed: Biological Citizens after Chernobyl*. Princeton, NJ: Princeton University Press.

Podlashuc, L. 2006. 'Class for Itself? Shack/Slum Dwellers International: The Praxis of a Transnational Urban Poor Movement'. Doctoral thesis, Faculty of Humanities and Social Sciences, University of Technology, Sydney.

Povinelli, E.A. 1999a. 'Settler Modernity and the Quest for Indigenous Tradition', *Public Culture* 11, 1: 19–48.

— 1999b. 'Consuming Geist: Popontology and the Spirit of Capital in Indigenous Australia', *Public Culture* 11, 1: 501–28.

Putnam, R. 1993. *Making Democracy Work: Civic Traditions in Modern Italy*. Princeton, NJ: Princeton University Press.

Rajan, K.S. 2006. *Biocapital: The Constitution of Postgenomic Life*. Durham, NC and London: Duke University Press.

Rassool, Ciraj, 1999. 'Cultural Performance and Fictions in Identity: the Case of the Khoisan of the Southern Kalahari, 1936–1937', in Y. Dladla (ed.) *Voices, Values and Identities Symposium*. Pretoria: South African National Parks.

Reid G. and Walker, L. (eds) 2005. *Men Behaving Differently: South African Men Since 1994*. Cape Town: Double Storey Publishers.

Reynolds Whyte, S. 2002. 'Subjectivity and Subjunctivity: Hoping for Health in Eastern Uganda', in R. Werbner (ed.) *Postcolonial Subjectivities in Africa*. London and New York: Zed Books.

Richter, L. and Morrell, R. (eds) 2006. *Baba: Men and Fatherhood in South Africa*. Cape Town: HSRC Press.

Robins, S. 1994. 'Contesting the Social Geometry of State Power: A Case Study of Land–Use Planning in Matabeleland, Zimbabwe', *Social Dynamics*, 20(2): 91–118.

— 1997. 'Transgressing the Borderlands of Tradition and Modernity: "Coloured" Identity, Cultural Hybridity and Land Struggles in Namaqualand (1980–94)', *Journal for Contemporary African Studies*, 15(1): 23–44.

— 1998. 'Bodies out of Place: Crossroads and Landscapes of Exclusion', in Juden, H. (ed.) *Blank: Interrogating Architecture After Apartheid*. Rotterdam: Netherlands Architectural Institute, pp. 457–70.

— 2000. 'Land Struggles and the Politics and Ethics of Representing "Bushman" History and Identity', *Kronos: Journal of Cape History, University of Western Cape*, 26: 56–75.

— 2002. 'At the Limits of Spatial Governmentality: A Message from the Tip of Africa', *Third World Quarterly* 23(4).

— 2003a. 'Grounding "Globalisation from Below": Global Citizens in Local Spaces', in Chidester, D., Dexter, P. and James, W. (eds) *What Holds Us Together: Social Cohesion in South Africa*. Cape Town: HSRC Publishers.

— 2003b. 'The Return of Ethnographic Authority? Comment on Adam Kuper's "The Return of the Native"', *Current Anthropology*, 44(3).

— 2003c. 'Reclaiming Bodies, Extending Citizenship: Health Activism in a Time of AIDS'. Unpublished paper, Association of Anthropology in Southern Africa conference, University of Cape Town, 24–7 August.

— 2004. '"Long Live Zackie, Long Live": AIDS Activism, Science and Citizenship after Apartheid', *Journal of Southern African Studies* 30(3): 651–72.

— (ed.) 2005a. *Limits to Liberation after Apartheid: Citizenship, Governance and Culture*. Oxford: James Currey.

— 2005b. 'The Politics of Ambiguity in a Time of AIDS', *Sunday Independent*, 6 March.

— 2006. 'From Rights to "Ritual": AIDS Activism and Treatment Testimonies in South Africa', *American Anthropologist* 108(2): 312–23.

Roitman, J. 2004. 'Productivity in the Margins: The Reconstruction of State Power in the Chad Basin', in Das, V. and Poole, D. (eds) *Anthropology in the Margins of the State*. Sante Fe: School of American Research Press and Oxford: James Currey.

Rose, N. 2007. *The Politics of Life Itself: Biomedicine, Power, and Subjectivity in the Twenty-First Century*. Princeton, NJ, and Oxford: Princeton University Press.

Rose, N. and Novas, C. 2005. 'Biological Citizenship', in Ong, A. and Collier, S.J. (eds) *Global Assemblages: Technology, Politics, and Ethics as Anthropological Problems*. Oxford: Blackwell Publishing.

Sachs, W. (ed.) 1992. *The Development Dictionary: A Guide to Knowledge and Power*. London: Zed Books.

Sahlins, M. 1999. 'What is Anthropological Enlightenment? Some Lessons of the Twentieth Century', *Annual Review of Anthropology* 28: i–xxiii.

Sampson, S. 1996. 'The social life of projects: imposing civil society to Albania', in Hann, C. and Dunn, E. (eds) *Civil Society: Challenging Western Models*. London and New York: Routledge.

Scott, J. 1998. *Seeing like a State: How Certain Schemes to Improve the Human Condition Have Failed*. New Haven, CT: Yale University Press.

Serematakis. C. 1991. *The Last Word. Women, Death and Divination in Inner Mani*. Chicago: Chicago University Press.

Sharp, J. 1977. 'Rural Development Schemes and the Struggle against Impoverishment in the Namaqualand Reserves'. Paper presented to the Second Carnegie Conference on Poverty and Development in South Africa, University of Cape Town.

— 1994. 'Land Claims in the Komaggas Reserve', *Review of African Political Economy*, 61: 403–14.

— 1996. 'Ethnogenesis and Ethnic Mobilization: A comparative perspective on a South African dilemma', in Wilson, E.N. and McAllister, P. (eds) *The Politics of Difference: Ethnic Premises in a World of Power*. Chicago and London: University of Chicago Press.

Sharp, J. and Douglas, S. 1996. 'Prisoners of their Reputation? The Veterans of the "Bushman" Battalions in South Africa', in Skotnes, P. (ed.) *Miscast: Negotiating the Presence of the Bushmen*. Cape Town: University of Cape Town Press.

Shepherd, N. and Robins, S. (eds) *New South African Keywords: A Concise Guide to Public and Political Discourse in Post-Apartheid Society*. Jacana (in press).

Shoepf, Brooke G. 2001. 'International AIDS Research in Anthropology: Taking a Critical Perspective on the Crisis', *Annual Review of Anthropology*, 30: 336.

Silberschmidt, M. 2005. 'Poverty, Male Disempowerment, and Male Sexuality: Rethinking Men and Masculinities in Rural and Urban East Africa', in Ouzgane, L. and Morrell, R. (eds) *African Masculinities: Men in Africa from the Late Nineteenth Century to the Present*. Basingstoke: Palgrave and Durban: University of Kwa-Zulu Natal Press.

Singer, L. 1990. *Erotic Welfare: Sexual Theory and Politics in the Age of Epidemic.* New York and London: Routledge.

Skotnes, P. (ed.) 1996. *Miscast: Negotiating the Presence of the Bushmen.* Cape Town: University of Cape Town Press.

Slum Dwellers International (SDI). 2002. *Journal* No. 2, March, Cape Town.

Spiegel, M. 1995. 'Migration, Urbanisation and Domestic Fluidity: Reviewing Some South African Examples', *African Anthropology*, II(2): 90–113.

Spivak, G. 1988. *In Other Worlds.* New York: Routledge.

Steyn, L. 1989. 'Dis Ons Land Maar Dis Nie Ons Land Nie: Dispossession of Land in Namaqualand', *Surplus People Project Report*, Cape Town.

Steyn, L. and Krohne, H. 1989. 'Land Use in Namaqualand', *Surplus People Project Report*, Cape Town.

Terreblanche, S. 2002. *A History of Inequality in South Africa 1652–2002.* Pietermaritzburg: University of Natal Press.

Touraine, Alain, 1974. *The Post-Industrial Society: Tomorrow's Social History: Classes, Conflicts and Culture in the Programmed Society.* New York: Random House.

— 1981. *The Voice and the Eye: An Analysis of Social Movements.* Cambridge: Cambridge University Press.

— 1985. 'An Introduction to the Study of New Social Movements', *Social Research* 52(4): 749–87.

Treichler, P. 1999. *How to have Theory in an Epidemic: Cultural Chronicles and AIDS.* Durham, NC: Duke University Press.

Turner, B.S. 1992. *Regulating Bodies: Essays in Medical Sociology.* London: Routledge.

Turner, V. 1957. *Schism and Continuity in an African Society.* Manchester: Manchester University Press, for the Rhodes-Livingstone Institute.

— 1961. *Ndembu Divination: Its Symbolism and Techniques.* Manchester: Manchester University Press.

— 1968. *The Drums of Affliction.* Oxford: Clarendon Press.

— 1969. *The Ritual Process: Structure and Anti-Structure.* Chicago: Aldine Publishing Company.

Van Gennep, A. 1960. *The Rites of Passage* (Translated by Monika B. Vizedom and Gabrielle L. Caffee.) London: Routledge and Kegan Paul.

Von Lieres, B. 2005. 'Marginalisation and Citizenship in Post-Apartheid South Africa', in Robins, S. (ed.) *Limits to Liberation after Apartheid: Citizenship, Governance and Culture.* Oxford: James Currey; Athens, OH: University of Ohio Press, and Cape Town: David Philip.

Wacquant, L. 1993. 'Urban outcasts: stigma and division in the black American ghetto and the French urban periphery', *International Journal of Urban and Regional Research* 17(3): 365–83.

Wallace, A. 1956. 'Revitalization Movements', *American Anthropologist*, 58: 264–81.

Warren, K.B. 1998. *Indigenous Movements and their Critics: Pan-Maya Activism in Guatemala.* Princeton, NJ: Princeton University Press.

Wasserman, H. 2003. 'New Media in a New Democracy: An Exploration of the Potential of the Internet for Civil Society Groups in South Africa', in Sarikakis, K. and Thusssu, D. (eds) *Ideologies of the Internet.* London: Hampton Press.

Watson, V. 2003. 'Conflicting Rationalities: Implications for Planning Theory and

Ethics', *Planning Theory and Practice*, 4(4): 395–407.

Werbner, R. (ed.) 2002. *Postcolonial Subjectivities in Africa*. London and New York: Zed Books.

White, H. 1995. *In the Tradition of the Forefathers: Bushman Traditionality at Kagga Kamma*. Cape Town: University of Cape Town Press.

Wilmsen, E.N. 1989. *Land Filled with Flies: A Political Economy of the Kalahari*. Chicago and London: University of Chicago Press.

Wilson, E.N. and McAllister, P. (eds) 1996. *The Politics of Difference: Ethnic Premises in a World of Power*. Chicago and London: University of Chicago Press.

Wisborg, P. and Rohde, R. 2003. 'TRANCRAA: Contested tenure reform in Namaqualand commons'. Policy Brief 5. Cape Town: Programme for Land and Agrarian Studies (PLAAS), University of the Western Cape.

Wolf, E. 1955. 'Types of Latin American Peasantry: A Preliminary Discussion', *American Anthropologist* 57: 452–71.

— 1966. 'Kinship, Friendship and Patron–Client Relations in Complex Societies', in Banton, M. (ed.) *The Social Anthropology of Complex Societies*. ASA Monograph 4. London: Tavistock.

— 1982. *Europe and the People without History*. Berkeley: University of California Press.

Wood, K. and Jewkes, R. 2001. '"Dangerous" Love: Reflections on Violence among Xhosa Township Youth', in Morrell, R. (ed.) *Changing Men in Southern Africa*. London: Zed Books.

Index

186

www.ingramcontent.com/pod-product-compliance
Lightning Source LLC
Chambersburg PA
CBHW070839030726
47504CB00005B/1160